Introduction

Welcome to the **Galveston Diet Cookbook for Menopause**, a comprehensive culinary companion designed specifically to support women navigating the transformative journey of menopause. This pivotal phase in a woman's life brings about numerous changes, both physical and emotional, which often necessitate a shift in dietary habits to promote overall health and well-being.

Authored by Jacob, a seasoned expert in women's health and nutrition, this cookbook is the culmination of years of research, experience, and a deep understanding of the unique nutritional needs of menopausal women. Grounded in the principles of the Galveston Diet, renowned for its emphasis on hormone balance and inflammation reduction, this cookbook offers a treasure trove of delicious and nourishing recipes tailored to alleviate common menopausal symptoms and promote vitality.

Menopause is a natural transition marked by fluctuating hormone levels, which can manifest in a myriad of ways, from hot flashes and mood swings to weight gain and fatigue. Through the power of nutrition, we have the ability to mitigate these symptoms and optimize our health during this transformative time. The recipes featured in this cookbook are meticulously crafted to harness the healing properties of wholesome ingredients, rich in phytonutrients, antioxidants, and essential nutrients vital for hormonal balance and overall wellness.

Whether you're seeking relief from bothersome symptoms, aiming to manage your weight, or simply looking to embrace a healthier lifestyle, the Galveston Diet Cookbook for Menopause provides you with a diverse array of flavorful and satisfying dishes to support your journey. From vibrant salads and hearty soups to satisfying mains and decadent desserts, each recipe is thoughtfully curated to cater to your nutritional needs while tantalizing your taste buds.

Embrace this opportunity to nourish your body, revitalize your health, and reclaim your vitality with the **Galveston Diet Cookbook for Menopause** as your trusted guide. Let these recipes inspire you on your path to hormonal balance, wellness, and radiant living during this empowering phase of life.

1. Grilled salmon with steamed broccoli

Ingredients:
* 4 salmon fillets (about 6 ounces each)
* 1 tablespoon olive oil
* Salt and pepper to taste
* 1 lemon, thinly sliced
* 1 teaspoon garlic powder
* 1 teaspoon dried oregano
* 1 teaspoon dried thyme
* 1 teaspoon paprika
* 1 head of broccoli, cut into florets
* 2 tablespoons water
* Lemon wedges for serving

Instructions:

1. Preheat your grill to medium-high heat. If using an indoor grill pan, lightly grease it with olive oil.

2. Pat the salmon fillets dry with paper towels. Rub them with olive oil and season with salt and pepper to taste.

3. In a small bowl, mix together the garlic powder, dried oregano, dried thyme, and paprika. Rub this mixture evenly over the salmon fillets.

4. Place the lemon slices on top of the seasoned salmon fillets.

5. Place the salmon fillets on the preheated grill, skin-side down if they have skin. Grill for about 4-5 minutes per side, or until the salmon is cooked through and easily flakes with a fork. Cooking time may vary depending on the thickness of the fillets.

6. While the salmon is grilling, prepare the steamed broccoli. Place the broccoli florets in a microwave-safe dish. Add 2 tablespoons of water to the dish. Cover with a microwave-safe lid or plastic wrap, leaving a small vent for steam to escape.

7. Microwave the broccoli on high for 3-4 minutes, or until tender but still crisp.

8. Serve the grilled salmon with steamed broccoli on the side. Squeeze fresh lemon juice over the salmon and broccoli before serving.

This dish is rich in omega-3 fatty acids from the salmon, which can help reduce inflammation associated with menopause. Broccoli is also a great source of nutrients like vitamins C and K, as well as fiber, which can support overall health during menopause.

2. Quinoa salad with roasted vegetables

Ingredients:

- 1 cup quinoa, rinsed
- 2 cups water or vegetable broth
- 1 red bell pepper, diced
- 1 yellow bell pepper, diced
- 1 zucchini, diced
- 1 yellow squash, diced
- 1 red onion, diced
- 2 tablespoons olive oil
- Salt and pepper to taste
- 1 teaspoon garlic powder
- 1 teaspoon dried thyme
- 1 teaspoon dried oregano
- Juice of 1 lemon
- 2 tablespoons chopped fresh parsley
- Optional: crumbled feta cheese or goat cheese (for serving)

Instructions:

1. Preheat your oven to 400°F (200°C).

2. In a medium saucepan, combine the quinoa and water or vegetable broth. Bring to a boil over medium heat, then reduce the heat to low, cover, and simmer for about 15-20 minutes, or until the quinoa is cooked and the liquid is absorbed. Remove from heat and let it sit covered for 5 minutes, then fluff with a fork.

3. While the quinoa is cooking, prepare the roasted vegetables. Place the diced bell peppers, zucchini, yellow squash, and red onion on a large baking sheet. Drizzle with olive oil and toss to coat evenly. Season with salt, pepper, garlic powder, dried thyme, and dried oregano, and toss again to coat the vegetables evenly.

4. Roast the vegetables in the preheated oven for 20-25 minutes, or until they are tender and slightly caramelized, stirring halfway through cooking.

5. In a large bowl, combine the cooked quinoa and roasted vegetables. Add the lemon juice and chopped parsley, and toss gently to combine.

6. Taste and adjust seasoning as needed, adding more salt, pepper, or lemon juice if desired.

7. If using, sprinkle the crumbled feta cheese or goat cheese over the quinoa salad before serving.

8. Serve the quinoa salad warm or at room temperature as a delicious and nutritious main dish or side dish.

This quinoa salad is packed with fiber, vitamins, and minerals from the quinoa and roasted vegetables, making it an excellent choice for supporting overall health during menopause.

3. Turkey and vegetable stir-fry

Ingredients:

- 1 lb (450g) lean ground turkey
- 2 tablespoons olive oil
- 3 cloves garlic, minced
- 1 tablespoon ginger, minced
- 1 onion, thinly sliced
- 1 bell pepper, thinly sliced
- 2 cups broccoli florets
- 1 carrot, julienned
- 1 zucchini, sliced
- 1/4 cup low-sodium soy sauce or tamari
- 2 tablespoons rice vinegar
- 1 tablespoon honey or maple syrup (optional)
- 1 teaspoon sesame oil
- 2 green onions, chopped (for garnish)
- Sesame seeds (for garnish)
- Cooked brown rice or quinoa (for serving)

Instructions:

1. Heat 1 tablespoon of olive oil in a large skillet or wok over medium-high heat. Add the ground turkey and cook, breaking it up with a spatula, until it is browned and cooked through. Remove the turkey from the skillet and set aside.

2. In the same skillet, add the remaining tablespoon of olive oil. Add the minced garlic and ginger, and cook for 1-2 minutes until fragrant.

3. Add the sliced onion and bell pepper to the skillet. Stir-fry for 2-3 minutes until they start to soften.

4. Add the broccoli florets, julienned carrot, and sliced zucchini to the skillet. Stir-fry for another 3-4 minutes until the vegetables are tender-crisp.

5. Return the cooked ground turkey to the skillet with the vegetables.

6. In a small bowl, whisk together the low-sodium soy sauce or tamari, rice vinegar, honey or maple syrup (if using), and sesame oil. Pour the sauce over the turkey and vegetables in the skillet.

7. Stir everything together until well combined and heated through, about 2-3 minutes.

8. Taste the stir-fry and adjust the seasoning if needed, adding more soy sauce or salt if desired.

9. Serve the turkey and vegetable stir-fry hot, garnished with chopped green onions and sesame seeds, over cooked brown rice or quinoa.

This turkey and vegetable stir-fry is loaded with lean protein and colorful vegetables, providing essential nutrients and supporting overall health during menopause.

4. Greek yogurt with berries and almonds

Here's a simple and nutritious recipe for Greek Yogurt with Berries and Almonds, suitable for the Galveston Diet, which emphasizes whole, anti-inflammatory foods beneficial for menopause:

Ingredients:
- 1 cup Greek yogurt (plain, unsweetened)
- 1/2 cup mixed berries (such as strawberries, blueberries, raspberries)
- 2 tablespoons sliced almonds
- 1 tablespoon honey or maple syrup (optional, for sweetness)
- A sprinkle of cinnamon (optional, for extra flavor)

Instructions:

1. Start by spooning the Greek yogurt into a serving bowl or individual serving cups.

2. Rinse the mixed berries under cold water and pat them dry with a paper towel. If using strawberries, hull and slice them.

3. Arrange the mixed berries on top of the Greek yogurt. Sprinkle the sliced almonds over the berries and yogurt.

4. If desired, drizzle the honey or maple syrup over the yogurt and berries for a touch of sweetness.

5. Optional: Finish with a sprinkle of cinnamon for extra flavor. Serve immediately and enjoy this nutritious and delicious Greek yogurt with berries and almonds as a satisfying snack or light breakfast.

This recipe provides a good balance of protein, healthy fats, and fiber-rich carbohydrates, making it an excellent choice for supporting overall health during menopause. The Greek yogurt offers probiotics for gut health, while berries provide antioxidants and almonds offer healthy fats and crunch.

5. Lentil soup with spinach

Ingredients:
- 1 cup dried green or brown lentils, rinsed and picked over
- 1 tablespoon olive oil
- 1 onion, chopped
- 2 carrots, chopped
- 2 celery stalks, chopped
- 3 cloves garlic, minced
- 1 teaspoon ground cumin
- 1 teaspoon ground coriander
- 1/2 teaspoon smoked paprika
- 6 cups vegetable broth or water
- 1 can (14 ounces) diced tomatoes, with juices
- 2 cups fresh spinach leaves, chopped
- Salt and pepper to taste
- Fresh lemon wedges, for serving (optional)

Instructions:

1. In a large pot or Dutch oven, heat the olive oil over medium heat. Add the chopped onion, carrots, and celery. Cook, stirring occasionally, until the vegetables are softened, about 5-7 minutes.

2. Add the minced garlic, ground cumin, ground coriander, and smoked paprika to the pot. Cook, stirring constantly, for 1-2 minutes until fragrant.

3. Add the rinsed lentils, vegetable broth or water, and diced tomatoes with their juices to the pot. Stir to combine.

4. Bring the soup to a boil, then reduce the heat to low. Cover and simmer for 25-30 minutes, or until the lentils are tender.

5. Once the lentils are cooked, stir in the chopped spinach leaves. Cook for an additional 2-3 minutes until the spinach is wilted.

6. Taste the soup and season with salt and pepper to taste.

7. Ladle the lentil soup into bowls and serve hot, with fresh lemon wedges on the side for squeezing over the soup, if desired.

8. Enjoy this hearty and nutritious lentil soup with spinach as a comforting meal that's perfect for supporting overall health during menopause.

This lentil soup is rich in fiber, protein, vitamins, and minerals, making it an excellent choice for menopausal women following the Galveston Diet. The spinach adds a boost of iron and other essential nutrients.

6. Chicken salad with avocado

Ingredients:

- 2 cups cooked chicken breast, diced or shredded
- 1 ripe avocado, diced
- 1/4 cup red onion, finely chopped
- 1/4 cup celery, finely chopped
- 1/4 cup Greek yogurt (plain, unsweetened)
- 1 tablespoon fresh lemon juice
- 1 tablespoon chopped fresh cilantro or parsley
- Salt and pepper to taste
- Lettuce leaves or mixed greens, for serving

Instructions:

1. In a large mixing bowl, combine the diced chicken breast, diced avocado, chopped red onion, and chopped celery.

2. In a small bowl, whisk together the Greek yogurt and fresh lemon juice until smooth.

3. Pour the Greek yogurt mixture over the chicken and avocado mixture in the large bowl. Add the chopped cilantro or parsley, and season with salt and pepper to taste.

4. Gently toss all the ingredients together until well combined and evenly coated with the yogurt dressing.

5. Serve the chicken salad on a bed of lettuce leaves or mixed greens. Enjoy this delicious and satisfying chicken salad with avocado as a nutritious meal that's perfect for supporting overall health during menopause.

This recipe provides lean protein from the chicken, healthy fats from the avocado, and plenty of vitamins and minerals from the vegetables, making it an excellent choice for menopausal women following the Galveston Diet.

7. Tofu and vegetable curry

Ingredients:
- 1 block (14 oz) firm tofu, drained and cubed
- 2 tablespoons olive oil or coconut oil
- 1 onion, chopped
- 3 cloves garlic, minced
- 1 tablespoon fresh ginger, grated
- 2 tablespoons curry powder
- 1 teaspoon ground turmeric
- 1 teaspoon ground cumin
- 1 can (14 oz) coconut milk
- 1 teaspoon ground coriander
- 1 cup vegetable broth
- 2 cups mixed vegetables (such as bell peppers, broccoli, carrots, snap peas)
- Salt and pepper to taste
- Cooked brown rice or quinoa, for serving
- Fresh cilantro leaves, for garnish (optional)
- Lime wedges, for serving (optional)

Instructions:
1. Heat 1 tablespoon of olive oil or coconut oil in a large skillet or Dutch oven over medium heat. Add the cubed tofu and cook until golden brown on all sides, about 5-7 minutes. Remove the tofu from the skillet and set aside.

2. In the same skillet, add the remaining tablespoon of oil. Add the chopped onion and cook until softened, about 5 minutes.

3. Add the minced garlic and grated ginger to the skillet. Cook for an additional 1-2 minutes until fragrant.

4. Stir in the curry powder, ground turmeric, ground cumin, and ground coriander. Cook for 1 minute until the spices are toasted and aromatic.

5. Pour in the coconut milk and vegetable broth. Stir to combine, scraping up any browned bits from the bottom of the skillet.

6. Add the mixed vegetables to the skillet. Bring the mixture to a simmer and cook for 8-10 minutes, or until the vegetables are tender.

7. Return the cooked tofu to the skillet. Stir gently to combine and heat through.

8. Season the curry with salt and pepper to taste. Serve the tofu and vegetable curry hot, over cooked brown rice or quinoa.

9. Garnish with fresh cilantro leaves and serve with lime wedges on the side, if desired.

Enjoy this flavorful and nutritious tofu and vegetable curry as a satisfying meal that's perfect for supporting overall health during menopause. This recipe provides plant-based protein from the tofu, a variety of colorful vegetables rich in vitamins and minerals, and anti-inflammatory spices like turmeric, making it an excellent choice for menopausal women following the Galveston Diet.

8. Shrimp and vegetable skewers

Ingredients:
- 2 tablespoons olive oil
- 2 cloves garlic, minced
- 1 teaspoon smoked paprika
- 1 teaspoon dried oregano
- 1/2 teaspoon ground cumin
- Salt and pepper to taste
- 1 red bell pepper, cut into chunks
- 1 yellow bell pepper, cut into chunks
- 1 red onion, cut into chunks
- 1 zucchini, sliced into rounds
- Wooden or metal skewers
- 1 lb (450g) large shrimp, peeled and deveined

Instructions:
1. If using wooden skewers, soak them in water for at least 30 minutes to prevent them from burning during cooking.

2. In a large bowl, combine the peeled and deveined shrimp with olive oil, minced garlic, smoked paprika, dried oregano, ground cumin, salt, and pepper. Toss until the shrimp are evenly coated with the seasonings. Marinate in the refrigerator for at least 15 minutes, or up to 1 hour.

3. Preheat your grill to medium-high heat.

4. Thread the marinated shrimp, chunks of bell pepper, onion, and slices of zucchini onto the skewers, alternating between shrimp and vegetables.

5. Lightly oil the grill grates to prevent sticking. Place the skewers on the preheated grill.

6. Grill the skewers for 2-3 minutes on each side, or until the shrimp are pink and opaque and the vegetables are tender-crisp, with a slight char.

7. Remove the skewers from the grill and transfer them to a serving platter.

8. Serve the shrimp and vegetable skewers hot, with your choice of side dishes or dipping sauces.

Enjoy these delicious and nutritious shrimp and vegetable skewers as a satisfying meal that's perfect for supporting overall health during menopause.

This recipe provides lean protein from the shrimp, along with a variety of colorful vegetables rich in vitamins, minerals, and antioxidants, making it an excellent choice for menopausal women following the Galveston Diet.

9. Spinach and feta omelet

Ingredients:
- 3 large eggs
- 1 tablespoon water or milk
- Salt and pepper to taste
- 1 teaspoon olive oil or butter
- 1 cup fresh spinach leaves
- 2 tablespoons crumbled feta cheese

Instructions:

1. In a small bowl, whisk together the eggs, water or milk, salt, and pepper until well combined.

2. Heat the olive oil or butter in a non-stick skillet over medium heat.

3. Add the fresh spinach leaves to the skillet and cook for 1-2 minutes, stirring occasionally, until wilted. Spread the spinach evenly across the bottom of the skillet.

4. Pour the whisked egg mixture over the spinach in the skillet, swirling gently to spread it out evenly.

5. Cook the omelet for 2-3 minutes, or until the edges begin to set and the bottom is lightly golden brown. Sprinkle the crumbled feta cheese evenly over one half of the omelet.

6. Using a spatula, carefully fold the other half of the omelet over the side with the cheese, creating a half-moon shape.

7. Cook for an additional 1-2 minutes, or until the cheese is melted and the omelet is cooked through to your liking. Slide the spinach and feta omelet onto a plate and serve hot.

Enjoy this flavorful and nutritious spinach and feta omelet as a satisfying meal that's perfect for supporting overall health during menopause.

This recipe provides protein and essential nutrients from the eggs, along with the antioxidant-rich spinach and calcium-rich feta cheese, making it an excellent choice for menopausal women following the Galveston Diet. Enjoy!

10. Whole grain pasta with marinara sauce

Ingredients:
- 8 ounces whole grain pasta (such as whole wheat or brown rice pasta)
- 1 tablespoon olive oil
- 1 onion, chopped
- 2 cloves garlic, minced
- 1 can (28 ounces) crushed tomatoes
- 1 teaspoon dried basil
- 1 teaspoon dried oregano
- 1/2 teaspoon dried thyme
- Salt and pepper to taste
- Optional toppings: Fresh basil leaves, grated Parmesan cheese

Instructions:

1. Cook the whole grain pasta according to the package instructions until al dente. Drain and set aside.

2. In a large skillet, heat the olive oil over medium heat. Add the chopped onion and cook until softened, about 5 minutes.

3. Add the minced garlic to the skillet and cook for an additional 1-2 minutes until fragrant.

4. Stir in the crushed tomatoes, dried basil, dried oregano, dried thyme, salt, and pepper. Bring the sauce to a simmer.

5. Reduce the heat to low and let the sauce simmer for 15-20 minutes, stirring occasionally, to allow the flavors to meld and the sauce to thicken slightly.

6. Taste the marinara sauce and adjust the seasoning as needed, adding more salt, pepper, or herbs if desired.

7. Once the sauce is ready, toss the cooked whole grain pasta with the marinara sauce until well coated.

8. Serve the whole grain pasta with marinara sauce hot, garnished with fresh basil leaves and grated Parmesan cheese if desired.

Enjoy this delicious and satisfying whole grain pasta with marinara sauce as a comforting meal that's perfect for supporting overall health during menopause.

This recipe provides complex carbohydrates from the whole grain pasta, along with the antioxidant-rich tomatoes and herbs, making it an excellent choice for menopausal women following the Galveston Diet.

11. Roasted chicken with sweet potatoes

Ingredients:
- 4 bone-in, skin-on chicken thighs (or any preferred chicken pieces)
- 2 medium sweet potatoes, peeled and cut into chunks
- 2 tablespoons olive oil
- 2 cloves garlic, minced
- 1 teaspoon dried thyme
- 1 teaspoon dried rosemary
- Salt and pepper to taste
- Optional: chopped fresh parsley for garnish

Instructions:

1. Preheat your oven to 400°F (200°C).

2. In a small bowl, mix together the olive oil, minced garlic, dried thyme, dried rosemary, salt, and pepper.

3. Place the chicken thighs and sweet potato chunks on a large baking sheet or roasting pan.

4. Drizzle the olive oil mixture over the chicken thighs and sweet potatoes. Use your hands or a spoon to toss everything together until evenly coated with the seasoning.

5. Arrange the chicken thighs skin-side up on the baking sheet, making sure they are not overcrowded. Spread the sweet potato chunks around the chicken.

6. Roast in the preheated oven for 35-40 minutes, or until the chicken is cooked through and the sweet potatoes are tender, flipping the chicken halfway through cooking.

7. Once the chicken is cooked and the sweet potatoes are tender, remove the baking sheet from the oven.

8. Optional: Garnish with chopped fresh parsley before serving.

9. Serve the roasted chicken thighs and sweet potatoes hot, as a delicious and satisfying meal that's perfect for supporting overall health during menopause.

This recipe provides lean protein from the chicken thighs and complex carbohydrates from the sweet potatoes, making it an excellent choice for menopausal women following the Galveston Diet. Enjoy!

12. Bean and vegetable chili

Ingredients:
- 1 tablespoon olive oil
- 1 onion, chopped
- 3 cloves garlic, minced
- 1 bell pepper, diced
- 2 carrots, diced
- 2 stalks celery, diced
- 1 zucchini, diced
- 1 yellow squash, diced
- 1 can (14 ounces) diced tomatoes
- 2 cans (14 ounces each) kidney beans, drained and rinsed
- 2 cups vegetable broth
- 2 tablespoons chili powder
- 1 teaspoon ground cumin
- 1 teaspoon smoked paprika
- Salt and pepper to taste
- Optional toppings: chopped fresh cilantro, diced avocado, shredded cheese, Greek yogurt or sour cream

Instructions:

1. Heat the olive oil in a large pot or Dutch oven over medium heat.

2. Add the chopped onion to the pot and cook until softened, about 5 minutes.

3. Add the minced garlic, diced bell pepper, diced carrots, diced celery, diced zucchini, and diced yellow squash to the pot. Cook, stirring occasionally, for 5-7 minutes, or until the vegetables start to soften.

4. Stir in the diced tomatoes, drained and rinsed kidney beans, vegetable broth, chili powder, ground cumin, smoked paprika, salt, and pepper.

5. Bring the chili to a simmer, then reduce the heat to low. Cover and let it simmer for 20-30 minutes, stirring occasionally, to allow the flavors to meld and the vegetables to become tender.

6. Taste the chili and adjust the seasoning as needed, adding more salt, pepper, or spices to taste.

7. Serve the bean and vegetable chili hot, garnished with your choice of toppings such as chopped fresh cilantro, diced avocado, shredded cheese, or Greek yogurt/sour cream.

8. Enjoy this flavorful and nutritious bean and vegetable chili as a comforting meal that's perfect for supporting overall health during menopause.

This recipe provides plant-based protein from the kidney beans, along with a variety of colorful vegetables rich in vitamins, minerals, and antioxidants, making it an excellent choice for menopausal women following the Galveston Diet.

13. Greek salad with grilled chicken

Ingredients:
For the Greek Salad:
- 4 cups mixed salad greens
(such as romaine lettuce, spinach, and arugula)
- 1 cucumber, sliced
- 1 cup cherry tomatoes, halved
- 1/2 red onion, thinly sliced
- 1/2 cup Kalamata olives, pitted
- 1/2 cup crumbled feta cheese

- 2 tablespoons chopped fresh parsley
- 2 tablespoons extra-virgin olive oil
- 1 tablespoon red wine vinegar
- 1 teaspoon dried oregano
- Salt and pepper to taste
- Lemon wedges, for serving

For the Grilled Chicken:
- 4 boneless, skinless chicken breasts
- 2 tablespoons olive oil
- 2 cloves garlic, minced
- 1 teaspoon dried oregano
- Salt and pepper to taste

Instructions:
1. Preheat your grill to medium-high heat.

2. In a small bowl, mix together the olive oil, minced garlic, dried oregano, salt, and pepper. Rub this mixture evenly over the chicken breasts.

3. Place the seasoned chicken breasts on the preheated grill. Grill for 6-8 minutes per side, or until the chicken is cooked through and no longer pink in the center. Cooking time may vary depending on the thickness of the chicken breasts. Once cooked, remove the chicken from the grill and let it rest for a few minutes before slicing.

4. While the chicken is grilling, prepare the Greek salad. In a large salad bowl, combine the mixed salad greens, sliced cucumber, halved cherry tomatoes, thinly sliced red onion, Kalamata olives, crumbled feta cheese, and chopped fresh parsley.

5. In a small bowl, whisk together the extra-virgin olive oil, red wine vinegar, dried oregano, salt, and pepper to make the dressing.

6. Drizzle the dressing over the Greek salad and toss gently to combine. Divide the Greek salad evenly among serving plates.

7. Slice the grilled chicken breasts and arrange them on top of the Greek salad.

8. Serve the Greek salad with grilled chicken immediately, with lemon wedges on the side for squeezing over the chicken if desired.

Enjoy this delicious and nutritious Greek salad with grilled chicken as a satisfying meal that's perfect for supporting overall health during menopause.

This recipe provides lean protein from the grilled chicken, along with a variety of colorful vegetables rich in vitamins, minerals, and antioxidants, making it an excellent choice for menopausal women following the Galveston Diet.

14. Oatmeal topped with nuts and fruits

Ingredients:
- 1/2 cup old-fashioned rolled oats
- 1 cup water or milk of your choice (such as almond milk, coconut milk, or dairy milk)
- Pinch of salt
- 1/4 teaspoon ground cinnamon (optional)
- 1/4 cup mixed nuts (such as almonds, walnuts, pecans)
- 1/4 cup mixed fresh or dried fruits (such as berries, sliced banana, diced apple, raisins, dried cranberries)
- Drizzle of honey or maple syrup (optional, for sweetness)
- Additional toppings as desired (such as chia seeds, flaxseeds, coconut flakes)

Instructions:

1. In a small saucepan, combine the rolled oats, water or milk, salt, and ground cinnamon (if using). Stir to combine.

2. Place the saucepan over medium heat and bring the mixture to a gentle boil.

3. Reduce the heat to low and simmer the oatmeal, stirring occasionally, for about 5-7 minutes or until the oats are cooked and the mixture has thickened to your desired consistency.

4. While the oatmeal is cooking, roughly chop the mixed nuts.

5. Once the oatmeal is cooked, remove the saucepan from the heat and transfer the oatmeal to a serving bowl.

6. Top the oatmeal with the chopped mixed nuts and mixed fruits.

7. If desired, drizzle the oatmeal with honey or maple syrup for a touch of sweetness.

8. Add any additional toppings you like, such as chia seeds, flaxseeds, or coconut flakes.

9. Serve the oatmeal topped with nuts and fruits hot, and enjoy this nutritious and satisfying breakfast that's perfect for supporting overall health during menopause.

This recipe provides complex carbohydrates, fiber, and essential nutrients from the oats, along with healthy fats, protein, and additional nutrients from the nuts and fruits, making it an excellent choice for menopausal women following the Galveston Diet. Enjoy!

15. Veggie burger with a side salad

Veggie Burger Ingredients:
- 1 can (15 ounces) chickpeas, drained and rinsed
- 1 cup cooked quinoa
- 1/2 cup old-fashioned oats
- 1/2 cup grated carrot
- 1/4 cup chopped red onion
- 2 cloves garlic, minced
- 2 tablespoons chopped fresh parsley
- 1 teaspoon ground cumin
- 1/2 teaspoon smoked paprika
- Salt and pepper to taste
- 1 tablespoon olive oil (for cooking)

Side Salad Ingredients:
- Mixed salad greens (such as spinach, arugula, and lettuce)
- Cherry tomatoes, halved
- Cucumber, sliced
- Red onion, thinly sliced
- Balsamic vinaigrette or dressing of your choice

Instructions:

1. In a food processor, combine the drained chickpeas, cooked quinoa, oats, grated carrot, chopped red onion, minced garlic, chopped fresh parsley, ground cumin, smoked paprika, salt, and pepper. Pulse until the mixture comes together but still has some texture.

2. Form the mixture into patties using your hands. If the mixture is too wet, you can add a little more oats to help bind it together.

3. Heat the olive oil in a large skillet over medium heat. Add the veggie burger patties to the skillet and cook for 4-5 minutes on each side, or until golden brown and heated through.

4. While the veggie burgers are cooking, prepare the side salad. In a large bowl, toss together the mixed salad greens, cherry tomatoes, sliced cucumber, and thinly sliced red onion.

5. Drizzle the salad with balsamic vinaigrette or dressing of your choice, and toss gently to coat.

6. Once the veggie burgers are cooked, serve them hot alongside the side salad.

7. Enjoy this nutritious and satisfying veggie burger with a side salad as a delicious meal that's perfect for supporting overall health during menopause.

This recipe provides plant-based protein, fiber, vitamins, and minerals from the chickpeas, quinoa, and vegetables, making it an excellent choice for menopausal women following the Galveston Diet.

16. Baked cod with asparagus

Ingredients:

- 4 cod fillets (about 6 ounces each)
- 1 bunch asparagus, tough ends trimmed
- 2 tablespoons olive oil
- 2 cloves garlic, minced
- 1 teaspoon lemon zest
- 1 tablespoon fresh lemon juice
- Salt and pepper to taste
- Optional: chopped fresh parsley or dill for garnish
- Lemon wedges, for serving

Instructions:

1. Preheat your oven to 400°F (200°C).

2. Place the asparagus spears on a large baking sheet. Drizzle with 1 tablespoon of olive oil and sprinkle with minced garlic. Toss to coat the asparagus evenly with the oil and garlic. Season with salt and pepper to taste.

3. Bake the asparagus in the preheated oven for 10-12 minutes, or until tender and lightly browned, shaking the pan halfway through cooking.

4. While the asparagus is baking, prepare the cod fillets. Pat the cod fillets dry with paper towels and place them on another baking sheet lined with parchment paper or aluminum foil.

5. In a small bowl, whisk together the remaining 1 tablespoon of olive oil, lemon zest, and lemon juice. Drizzle the mixture over the cod fillets and use a brush or spoon to spread it evenly.

6. Season the cod fillets with salt and pepper to taste.

7. Once the asparagus is done baking, remove it from the oven and set aside. Place the baking sheet with the cod fillets in the oven and bake for 12-15 minutes, or until the cod is opaque and flakes easily with a fork.

8. Serve the baked cod fillets alongside the roasted asparagus.

9. Garnish with chopped fresh parsley or dill, if desired, and serve with lemon wedges on the side for squeezing over the fish.

10. Enjoy this delicious and nutritious baked cod with asparagus as a satisfying meal that's perfect for supporting overall health during menopause.

This recipe provides lean protein from the cod, along with fiber, vitamins, and minerals from the asparagus, making it an excellent choice for menopausal women following the Galveston Diet.

17. Eggplant parmesan with whole grain bread

Ingredients:

For the Eggplant Parmesan:
- 1 large eggplant, sliced into 1/2-inch rounds
- 1 cup whole wheat breadcrumbs
- 1/2 cup grated Parmesan cheese
- 2 eggs, beaten
- 1 teaspoon dried oregano
- 1 teaspoon dried basil
- 1/2 teaspoon garlic powder
- Salt and pepper to taste
- Olive oil for frying
- 2 cups marinara sauce
- 1 cup shredded mozzarella cheese
- Fresh basil leaves for garnish (optional)

For the Whole Grain Bread: Whole grain bread slices

Instructions:

1. Preheat your oven to 375°F (190°C).

2. In a shallow dish, combine the whole wheat breadcrumbs, grated Parmesan cheese, dried oregano, dried basil, garlic powder, salt, and pepper.

3. Dip each eggplant slice into the beaten eggs, then coat it with the breadcrumb mixture, pressing gently to adhere. Repeat with all the eggplant slices.

4. Heat a thin layer of olive oil in a large skillet over medium heat. Working in batches, fry the breaded eggplant slices for 2-3 minutes on each side, or until golden brown and crispy. Add more olive oil to the skillet as needed for subsequent batches. Transfer the fried eggplant slices to a paper towel-lined plate to drain any excess oil.

5. In a baking dish, spread a thin layer of marinara sauce on the bottom. Arrange a layer of fried eggplant slices on top of the sauce. Spoon more marinara sauce over the eggplant slices, then sprinkle with shredded mozzarella cheese. Repeat the layers until all the eggplant slices are used, finishing with a layer of marinara sauce and mozzarella cheese on top.

6. Cover the baking dish with aluminum foil and bake in the preheated oven for 20-25 minutes, or until the cheese is melted and bubbly. While the eggplant Parmesan is baking, toast the whole grain bread slices.

7. Once the eggplant Parmesan is done baking, remove it from the oven and let it cool slightly before serving.

8. Serve the eggplant Parmesan hot, garnished with fresh basil leaves if desired, alongside the toasted whole grain bread slices.

9. Enjoy this delicious and nutritious eggplant Parmesan with whole grain bread as a satisfying meal that's perfect for supporting overall health during menopause.

This recipe provides fiber, vitamins, and minerals from the eggplant and whole grain bread, along with protein and calcium from the cheese, making it an excellent choice for menopausal women following the Galveston Diet. Enjoy!

18. Cottage cheese with pineapple

Ingredients:

- 1 cup cottage cheese (low-fat or full-fat, according to preference)
- 1 cup fresh pineapple chunks (or canned pineapple chunks in juice, drained)
- Optional: Honey or maple syrup for drizzling (if desired)

Instructions:

1. Spoon the cottage cheese into a serving bowl or individual serving cups.

2. Top the cottage cheese with the fresh pineapple chunks.

3. If desired, drizzle honey or maple syrup over the cottage cheese and pineapple for a touch of sweetness.

4. Serve immediately and enjoy this nutritious and delicious Cottage Cheese with Pineapple as a satisfying snack or light meal that's perfect for supporting overall health during menopause.

This recipe provides protein and calcium from the cottage cheese, along with vitamins, minerals, and antioxidants from the pineapple, making it an excellent choice for menopausal women following the Galveston Diet. Enjoy!

19. Vegetable frittata

Ingredients:

- 8 large eggs
- 1/4 cup milk (dairy or plant-based)
- Salt and pepper to taste
- 2 tablespoons olive oil
- 1 small onion, diced
- 1 bell pepper, diced
- 1 cup sliced mushrooms
- 1 cup baby spinach leaves
- 1 cup cherry tomatoes, halved
- 1/2 cup crumbled feta cheese (optional)
- 2 tablespoons chopped fresh herbs (such as parsley, basil, or chives)

Instructions

1. Preheat your oven to 350°F (175°C).

2. In a large mixing bowl, whisk together the eggs, milk, salt, and pepper until well combined. Set aside.

3. Heat the olive oil in an oven-safe skillet (such as a cast iron skillet) over medium heat.

4. Add the diced onion and diced bell pepper to the skillet. Cook, stirring occasionally, for 3-4 minutes, or until softened.

5. Add the sliced mushrooms to the skillet and cook for an additional 3-4 minutes, or until they start to brown.

6. Stir in the baby spinach leaves and cherry tomatoes, and cook for 1-2 minutes until the spinach is wilted and the tomatoes are softened. Spread the cooked vegetables evenly across the bottom of the skillet.

7. Pour the whisked egg mixture over the cooked vegetables in the skillet. Use a spatula to gently stir the mixture to distribute the vegetables evenly.

8. Sprinkle the crumbled feta cheese evenly over the top of the frittata mixture, if using.

9. Transfer the skillet to the preheated oven and bake for 20-25 minutes, or until the frittata is set and the top is lightly golden brown.

10. Once the frittata is cooked through, remove it from the oven and let it cool slightly. Sprinkle the chopped fresh herbs over the top of the frittata before slicing and serving.

11. Serve the vegetable frittata warm or at room temperature, sliced into wedges.

Enjoy this flavorful and nutritious Vegetable Frittata as a satisfying meal that's perfect for supporting overall health during menopause. This recipe provides protein, vitamins, and minerals from the eggs and a variety of colorful vegetables, making it an excellent choice for menopausal women following the Galveston Diet.

20. Black bean tacos with salsa

Ingredients:
For the Black Bean Filling:
- 1 tablespoon olive oil
- 1 small onion, diced
- 2 cloves garlic, minced
- 1 teaspoon ground cumin
- 1 teaspoon chili powder
- Salt and pepper to taste
- 1 tablespoon lime juice
- 2 tablespoons chopped fresh cilantro
- 1 can (15 ounces) black beans, drained and rinsed

For the Salsa:
- 1 cup diced tomatoes
- 1/4 cup diced red onion
- 1/4 cup chopped fresh cilantro
- 1 jalapeño pepper, seeded and finely chopped (optional, for heat)
- 1 tablespoon lime juice
- Salt and pepper to taste

For Serving:
- 8 small corn or whole wheat tortillas
- Optional toppings: sliced avocado, shredded lettuce, crumbled feta or queso fresco cheese, Greek yogurt or sour cream, lime wedges

Instructions:
1. To make the black bean filling, heat the olive oil in a skillet over medium heat. Add the diced onion and cook until softened, about 5 minutes.

2. Add the minced garlic, ground cumin, and chili powder to the skillet. Cook for 1-2 minutes until fragrant.

3. Stir in the drained and rinsed black beans. Cook for 5-7 minutes, mashing some of the beans with the back of a spoon, until heated through and the flavors are well combined.

4. Season the black bean filling with salt, pepper, lime juice, and chopped fresh cilantro. Stir to combine and keep warm while you prepare the salsa.

5. To make the salsa, combine the diced tomatoes, diced red onion, chopped fresh cilantro, finely chopped jalapeño pepper (if using), lime juice, salt, and pepper in a bowl. Stir to combine.

6. Warm the tortillas in a dry skillet or in the microwave according to package instructions.

7. To assemble the tacos, spoon the black bean filling onto each tortilla. Top with salsa and any desired toppings such as sliced avocado, shredded lettuce, crumbled cheese, and Greek yogurt or sour cream.

8. Serve the black bean tacos with salsa immediately, with lime wedges on the side for squeezing over the tacos if desired.

Enjoy these delicious and nutritious Black Bean Tacos with Salsa as a satisfying meal that's perfect for supporting overall health during menopause.

This recipe provides plant-based protein, fiber, vitamins, and minerals from the black beans and a variety of colorful vegetables, making it an excellent choice for menopausal women following the Galveston Diet.

21. Baked tofu with bok choy

Ingredients:
For the Baked Tofu:
- 1 block (14-16 ounces) extra-firm tofu
- 2 tablespoons soy sauce or tamari
- 1 tablespoon rice vinegar
- 1 tablespoon sesame oil
- 2 cloves garlic, minced
- 1 teaspoon grated ginger
- 1 tablespoon honey or maple syrup (optional, for sweetness)
- Salt and pepper to taste

For the Bok Choy:
- 4-6 baby bok choy, halved lengthwise
- 1 tablespoon olive oil
- 2 cloves garlic, minced
- Salt and pepper to taste

Instructions:
1. Preheat your oven to 400°F (200°C).

2. Press the tofu to remove excess water: Wrap the block of tofu in a clean kitchen towel or paper towels, then place it on a plate. Put a heavy object on top (such as a cast iron skillet or a couple of heavy cans) and let it sit for about 15-20 minutes.

3. While the tofu is pressing, prepare the marinade: In a small bowl, whisk together the soy sauce or tamari, rice vinegar, sesame oil, minced garlic, grated ginger, honey or maple syrup (if using), salt, and pepper.

4. Once the tofu has been pressed, unwrap it and cut it into cubes or slices, whichever you prefer.

5. Place the tofu pieces in a shallow dish or a zip-top bag. Pour the marinade over the tofu, making sure all pieces are coated evenly. Let it marinate for at least 15-20 minutes, or longer if time allows.

6. While the tofu is marinating, prepare the bok choy: In a large bowl, toss the halved bok choy with olive oil, minced garlic, salt, and pepper until evenly coated.

7. Arrange the marinated tofu pieces in a single layer on a baking sheet lined with parchment paper or aluminum foil. Bake in the preheated oven for 20-25 minutes, or until the tofu is golden brown and slightly crispy on the edges.

8. While the tofu is baking, place the prepared bok choy on another baking sheet. Roast in the oven for 10-12 minutes, or until the bok choy is tender and slightly charred.

9. Once the tofu and bok choy are cooked, remove them from the oven.

10. Serve the baked tofu with bok choy hot, garnished with sesame seeds or chopped green onions if desired.

Enjoy this flavorful and nutritious Baked Tofu with Bok Choy as a satisfying meal that's perfect for supporting overall health during menopause.

This recipe provides plant-based protein from the tofu, along with vitamins, minerals, and antioxidants from the bok choy, making it an excellent choice for menopausal women following the Galveston Diet.

22. Quinoa stuffed bell peppers

Ingredients:
- 4 large bell peppers, any color
- 1 cup quinoa, rinsed
- 2 cups vegetable broth or water
- 1 tablespoon olive oil
- 1 small onion, diced
- 2 cloves garlic, minced
- 1 carrot, diced
- 1 zucchini, diced
- 1 cup diced tomatoes (fresh or canned)
- 1 teaspoon dried oregano
- 1 teaspoon dried basil
- Salt and pepper to taste
- 1/2 cup shredded cheese (such as mozzarella or cheddar), optional
- Fresh parsley or basil for garnish, optional

Instructions:

1. Preheat your oven to 375°F (190°C).

2. Cut the tops off the bell peppers and remove the seeds and membranes. Place the hollowed-out bell peppers in a baking dish, cut side up. Set aside.

3. In a medium saucepan, combine the quinoa and vegetable broth or water. Bring to a boil, then reduce the heat to low, cover, and simmer for 15-20 minutes, or until the quinoa is cooked and the liquid is absorbed. Remove from heat and set aside.

4. In a large skillet, heat the olive oil over medium heat. Add the diced onion and cook until translucent, about 5 minutes.

5. Add the minced garlic, diced carrot, and diced zucchini to the skillet. Cook for an additional 5-7 minutes, or until the vegetables are tender.

6. Stir in the diced tomatoes, dried oregano, dried basil, salt, and pepper. Cook for 2-3 minutes more, until the mixture is heated through and fragrant.

7. Remove the skillet from heat and stir in the cooked quinoa. If desired, mix in the shredded cheese at this stage for added creaminess.

8. Spoon the quinoa and vegetable mixture evenly into the hollowed-out bell peppers.

9. Cover the baking dish with aluminum foil and bake in the preheated oven for 25-30 minutes, or until the bell peppers are tender.

10. Remove the foil and continue baking for an additional 5-10 minutes, or until the tops of the bell peppers are slightly browned.

11. Once cooked, remove the stuffed bell peppers from the oven and let them cool slightly.

12. Garnish with fresh parsley or basil, if desired, before serving.

Enjoy these flavorful and nutritious Quinoa Stuffed Bell Peppers as a satisfying meal that's perfect for supporting overall health during menopause.

This recipe provides complex carbohydrates, protein, fiber, vitamins, and minerals from the quinoa and a variety of colorful vegetables, making it an excellent choice for menopausal women following the Galveston Diet.

23. Turkey meatballs with zucchini noodles

Ingredients:
For the Turkey Meatballs:
- 1 lb ground turkey (preferably lean)
- 1/4 cup whole wheat breadcrumbs
- 1/4 cup grated Parmesan cheese
- 1 egg
- 2 cloves garlic, minced

- 1 teaspoon dried oregano
- 1 teaspoon dried basil
- Salt and pepper to taste
- Olive oil for cooking

For the Zucchini Noodles:
- 4 medium zucchini
- 2 tablespoons olive oil
- 2 cloves garlic, minced
- Salt and pepper to taste

Instructions:

1. Preheat your oven to 375°F (190°C).

2. In a large mixing bowl, combine the ground turkey, whole wheat breadcrumbs, grated Parmesan cheese, egg, minced garlic, dried oregano, dried basil, salt, and pepper. Mix until all ingredients are well combined.

3. Shape the turkey mixture into meatballs, about 1-1.5 inches in diameter.

4. Heat a small amount of olive oil in a large oven-safe skillet over medium heat. Add the turkey meatballs to the skillet and cook for 2-3 minutes on each side, until browned.

5. Once browned, transfer the skillet to the preheated oven and bake the meatballs for 15-20 minutes, or until they are cooked through and no longer pink in the center.

6. While the meatballs are baking, prepare the zucchini noodles. Using a spiralizer or a vegetable peeler, create zucchini noodles (also known as zoodles) from the zucchini.

7. Heat olive oil in a large skillet over medium heat. Add minced garlic and cook for about 1 minute until fragrant.

8. Add the zucchini noodles to the skillet and sauté for 2-3 minutes, or until they are just tender but still crisp. Season with salt and pepper to taste.

9. Once the turkey meatballs are cooked through, remove them from the oven. Serve the turkey meatballs over the zucchini noodles.

10. Optionally, garnish with fresh herbs like parsley or basil, and serve with marinara sauce or grated Parmesan cheese if desired.

Enjoy these flavorful and nutritious Turkey Meatballs with Zucchini Noodles as a satisfying meal that's perfect for supporting overall health during menopause. This recipe provides lean protein from the turkey meatballs, along with fiber, vitamins, and minerals from the zucchini noodles, making it an excellent choice for menopausal women following the Galveston Diet.

24. Greek yogurt parfait with granola

Ingredients:
- 1 cup Greek yogurt (low-fat or full-fat, according to preference)
- 1/2 cup granola (homemade or store-bought, choose one with low added sugars and whole grains)
- 1/2 cup mixed berries (such as strawberries, blueberries, raspberries)
- 1 tablespoon honey or maple syrup (optional, for sweetness)
- Optional toppings: sliced almonds, chopped walnuts, shredded coconut, chia seeds

Instructions:

1. In a serving glass or bowl, layer the Greek yogurt, granola, and mixed berries.

2. If desired, drizzle honey or maple syrup over the yogurt and berries for added sweetness.

3. Repeat the layers until the glass or bowl is filled, ending with a layer of granola on top.

4. Optionally, sprinkle additional toppings such as sliced almonds, chopped walnuts, shredded coconut, or chia seeds over the parfait for added texture and nutrition.

5. Serve the Greek yogurt parfait immediately, or cover and refrigerate for later enjoyment.

6. Enjoy this delicious and nutritious Greek Yogurt Parfait with Granola as a satisfying breakfast, snack, or dessert that's perfect for supporting overall health during menopause.

This recipe provides protein, probiotics, and calcium from the Greek yogurt, along with fiber, vitamins, and antioxidants from the granola and mixed berries, making it an excellent choice for menopausal women following the Galveston Diet. Enjoy!

25. Lentil and vegetable curry

Ingredients:
- 1 cup dry lentils (green or brown), rinsed and drained
- 2 tablespoons olive oil
- 1 onion, diced
- 2 cloves garlic, minced
- 1 tablespoon grated ginger
- 1 bell pepper, diced
- 2 carrots, diced
- 1 zucchini, diced
- 1 can (14 ounces) diced tomatoes
- 1 can (14 ounces) coconut milk
- 2 tablespoons curry powder
- 1 teaspoon ground cumin
- 1 teaspoon ground coriander
- 1/2 teaspoon turmeric
- Salt and pepper to taste
- Fresh cilantro for garnish (optional)
- Cooked brown rice or quinoa for serving

Instructions:

1. In a large pot or Dutch oven, heat the olive oil over medium heat. Add the diced onion and cook until softened, about 5 minutes.

2. Add the minced garlic and grated ginger to the pot. Cook for an additional 1-2 minutes until fragrant.

3. Stir in the diced bell pepper, carrots, and zucchini. Cook for 5-7 minutes until the vegetables start to soften.

4. Add the rinsed lentils, diced tomatoes (with their juices), and coconut milk to the pot. Stir to combine.

5. Season the mixture with curry powder, ground cumin, ground coriander, turmeric, salt, and pepper. Stir well to distribute the spices evenly.

6. Bring the curry to a simmer, then reduce the heat to low. Cover and let it simmer gently for 20-25 minutes, or until the lentils and vegetables are tender and the curry has thickened slightly. Stir occasionally to prevent sticking.

7. Taste the curry and adjust the seasoning if needed, adding more salt, pepper, or spices to taste.

8. Once the lentil and vegetable curry is cooked through and seasoned to your liking, remove it from the heat.

9. Serve the curry hot over cooked brown rice or quinoa. Garnish with fresh cilantro, if desired, before serving.

Enjoy this flavorful and nutritious Lentil and Vegetable Curry as a satisfying meal that's perfect for supporting overall health during menopause.

This recipe provides plant-based protein, fiber, vitamins, and minerals from the lentils and a variety of colorful vegetables, making it an excellent choice for menopausal women following the Galveston Diet.

26. Grilled steak with roasted Brussels sprouts

Ingredients:
For the Grilled Steak:
- 2 ribeye steaks, about 8 ounces each (or your preferred cut)
- 2 tablespoons olive oil
- 2 cloves garlic, minced
- 1 teaspoon dried thyme
- Salt and pepper to taste

For the Roasted Brussels Sprouts:
- 1 lb Brussels sprouts, trimmed and halved
- 2 tablespoons olive oil
- 2 cloves garlic, minced
- Salt and pepper to taste

Instructions:
1. Preheat your grill to medium-high heat.

2. In a small bowl, mix together the olive oil, minced garlic, dried thyme, salt, and pepper to create a marinade for the steak.

3. Pat the steaks dry with paper towels and then brush both sides of each steak with the marinade.

4. Place the steaks on the preheated grill and cook for about 4-5 minutes on each side for medium-rare, or longer if desired for your preferred level of doneness.

5. While the steaks are grilling, preheat your oven to 400°F (200°C) and prepare the Brussels sprouts.

6. In a large bowl, toss the halved Brussels sprouts with olive oil, minced garlic, salt, and pepper until evenly coated.

7. Spread the Brussels sprouts out in a single layer on a baking sheet lined with parchment paper.

8. Roast the Brussels sprouts in the preheated oven for 20-25 minutes, or until they are tender and golden brown, stirring halfway through cooking.

9. Once the steaks are done grilling to your liking, remove them from the grill and let them rest for a few minutes before slicing.

10. Serve the grilled steak slices with the roasted Brussels sprouts on the side. Optionally, garnish with chopped fresh herbs such as parsley or thyme before serving.

Enjoy this delicious and nutritious Grilled Steak with Roasted Brussels Sprouts as a satisfying meal that's perfect for supporting overall health during menopause.

This recipe provides protein and iron from the steak, along with fiber, vitamins, and antioxidants from the Brussels sprouts, making it an excellent choice for menopausal women following the Galveston Diet.

27. Chicken and vegetable kabobs

Ingredients:

For the Chicken:
- 1 lb boneless, skinless chicken breasts, cut into 1-inch cubes
- 2 tablespoons olive oil
- 2 cloves garlic, minced
- 1 teaspoon dried oregano
- 1 teaspoon paprika
- Salt and pepper to taste

For the Vegetable Kabobs:
- 1 bell pepper, cut into chunks
- 1 red onion, cut into chunks
- 1 zucchini, sliced into rounds
- 1 yellow squash, sliced into rounds
- 8-10 cherry tomatoes
- Wooden or metal skewers

Instructions:

1. If using wooden skewers, soak them in water for at least 30 minutes to prevent burning during grilling.

2. In a mixing bowl, combine the olive oil, minced garlic, dried oregano, paprika, salt, and pepper. Add the cubed chicken to the bowl and toss to coat the chicken evenly with the marinade. Cover the bowl and let the chicken marinate in the refrigerator for at least 30 minutes, or up to 4 hours.

3. Preheat your grill to medium-high heat.

4. Thread the marinated chicken cubes onto the skewers, alternating with the chunks of bell pepper, red onion, zucchini, yellow squash, and cherry tomatoes.

5. Brush the assembled kabobs with any remaining marinade from the bowl.

6. Place the kabobs on the preheated grill and cook for 10-12 minutes, turning occasionally, or until the chicken is cooked through and the vegetables are tender and slightly charred.

7. Once cooked, remove the kabobs from the grill and let them rest for a few minutes before serving.

8. Serve the chicken and vegetable kabobs hot, garnished with chopped fresh parsley or cilantro if desired.

Enjoy these flavorful and nutritious Chicken and Vegetable Kabobs as a satisfying meal that's perfect for supporting overall health during menopause.

This recipe provides lean protein from the chicken, along with fiber, vitamins, and minerals from the assortment of colorful vegetables, making it an excellent choice for menopausal women following the Galveston Diet.

28. Whole grain toast with avocado and tomato

Ingredients:
- 2 slices of whole grain bread
- 1 ripe avocado
- 1 medium tomato, sliced
- Salt and pepper to taste
- Optional toppings: red pepper flakes, sliced red onion, fresh herbs (such as basil or cilantro)

Instructions:

1. Toast the slices of whole grain bread until golden brown and crispy.

2. While the bread is toasting, prepare the avocado: Cut the avocado in half lengthwise, remove the pit, and scoop the flesh into a bowl. Use a fork to mash the avocado until smooth or leave it slightly chunky if desired. Season with salt and pepper to taste.

3. Once the bread is toasted, spread a generous amount of mashed avocado onto each slice. Top the avocado spread with slices of fresh tomato.

4. Season the tomato slices with a pinch of salt and pepper, and any additional toppings of your choice, such as red pepper flakes, sliced red onion, or fresh herbs. Serve the whole grain toast with avocado and tomato immediately.

Enjoy this delicious and nutritious Whole Grain Toast with Avocado and Tomato as a satisfying breakfast, snack, or light meal that's perfect for supporting overall health during menopause.

This recipe provides fiber, healthy fats, vitamins, and minerals from the whole grain bread, avocado, and tomato, making it an excellent choice for menopausal women following the Galveston Diet.

29. Stir-fried tofu with broccoli and carrots

Ingredients:
For the Stir-Fry Sauce:
- 3 tablespoons soy sauce
(or tamari for gluten-free option)
- 2 tablespoons rice vinegar
- 1 tablespoon honey or maple syrup
- 1 tablespoon sesame oil
- 2 cloves garlic, minced
- 1 teaspoon grated ginger
- 1 teaspoon cornstarch
(optional, for thickening)

For the Stir-Fry:
- 14-16 ounces firm tofu, pressed and cubed
- 2 tablespoons olive oil or vegetable oil
- 2 cups broccoli florets
- 2 medium carrots, julienned or thinly sliced
- Cooked brown rice or quinoa for serving
- Optional garnishes: sesame seeds, sliced green onions, chopped cilantro

Instructions:
1. In a small bowl, whisk together all the ingredients for the stir-fry sauce: soy sauce, rice vinegar, honey or maple syrup, sesame oil, minced garlic, grated ginger, and cornstarch (if using). Set aside.

2. Heat one tablespoon of oil in a large skillet or wok over medium-high heat. Add the cubed tofu and cook for 4-5 minutes, flipping occasionally, until golden brown and crispy on all sides. Remove tofu from the skillet and set aside.

3. In the same skillet, add another tablespoon of oil if needed. Add the broccoli florets and julienned carrots to the skillet. Stir-fry for 4-5 minutes, or until the vegetables are tender-crisp.

4. Return the cooked tofu to the skillet with the vegetables.

5. Pour the prepared stir-fry sauce over the tofu and vegetables in the skillet. Stir well to coat everything evenly with the sauce.

6. Cook for an additional 1-2 minutes, or until the sauce has thickened slightly and everything is heated through.

7. Remove the skillet from the heat. Serve the stir-fried tofu with broccoli and carrots over cooked brown rice or quinoa.

8. Garnish with sesame seeds, sliced green onions, and chopped cilantro, if desired.

Enjoy this flavorful and nutritious Stir-Fried Tofu with Broccoli and Carrots as a satisfying meal that's perfect for supporting overall health during menopause.

This recipe provides plant-based protein from the tofu, along with fiber, vitamins, and minerals from the broccoli and carrots, making it an excellent choice for menopausal women following the Galveston Diet.

30. Vegetable and bean soup

Ingredients:

- 2 tablespoons olive oil
- 1 onion, diced
- 2 cloves garlic, minced
- 2 carrots, diced
- 2 celery stalks, diced
- 1 bell pepper, diced
- 1 zucchini, diced
- 1 can (14 ounces) diced tomatoes
- 4 cups vegetable broth
- 2 cups water
- 1 can (15 ounces) cannellini beans, drained and rinsed
- 1 can (15 ounces) kidney beans, drained and rinsed
- 1 teaspoon dried oregano
- 1 teaspoon dried basil
- 1/2 teaspoon dried thyme
- Salt and pepper to taste
- 2 cups chopped spinach or kale
- Fresh parsley for garnish (optional)

Instructions:

1. In a large pot or Dutch oven, heat the olive oil over medium heat.

2. Add the diced onion, minced garlic, diced carrots, diced celery, diced bell pepper, and diced zucchini to the pot. Cook, stirring occasionally, for about 5-7 minutes until the vegetables are softened.

3. Stir in the diced tomatoes (with their juices), vegetable broth, water, cannellini beans, kidney beans, dried oregano, dried basil, dried thyme, salt, and pepper.

4. Bring the soup to a simmer, then reduce the heat to low. Cover and let the soup simmer gently for about 20-25 minutes to allow the flavors to meld together.

5. After simmering, taste the soup and adjust the seasoning with more salt and pepper if needed.

6. Stir in the chopped spinach or kale and cook for an additional 2-3 minutes until the greens are wilted.

7. Once the greens are wilted, remove the soup from the heat. Serve the vegetable and bean soup hot, garnished with fresh parsley if desired.

Enjoy this hearty and nutritious Vegetable and Bean Soup as a satisfying meal that's perfect for supporting overall health during menopause.

This recipe provides fiber, protein, vitamins, and minerals from the assortment of vegetables and beans, making it an excellent choice for menopausal women following the Galveston Diet.

31. Greek yogurt smoothie with spinach and banana

Ingredients:
- 1 ripe banana, peeled and sliced
- 1 cup fresh spinach leaves
- 1/2 cup Greek yogurt (low-fat or full-fat, according to preference)
- 1/2 cup unsweetened almond milk or any milk of your choice
- 1 tablespoon honey or maple syrup (optional, for added sweetness)
- 1/2 teaspoon vanilla extract
- Optional add-ins: chia seeds, flax seeds, protein powder, or nut butter for extra protein and nutrients
- Ice cubes (optional, for a colder smoothie)

Instructions:
1. Place the sliced banana, fresh spinach leaves, Greek yogurt, unsweetened almond milk, honey or maple syrup (if using), and vanilla extract in a blender.

2. If using any optional add-ins such as chia seeds, flax seeds, protein powder, or nut butter, add them to the blender as well.

3. If desired, add a handful of ice cubes to the blender to make the smoothie colder.

4. Blend all the ingredients until smooth and creamy, scraping down the sides of the blender as needed to ensure everything is well blended.

5. Taste the smoothie and adjust the sweetness or consistency by adding more honey, maple syrup, or almond milk if desired.

6. Once the smoothie reaches your desired consistency and sweetness, pour it into glasses and serve immediately.

7. Optionally, garnish the smoothie with a sprinkle of chia seeds, flax seeds, or sliced banana for added texture and presentation.

Enjoy this delicious and nutritious Greek Yogurt Smoothie with Spinach and Banana as a satisfying breakfast, snack, or post-workout drink that's perfect for supporting overall health during menopause.

This recipe provides protein, calcium, vitamins, and minerals from the Greek yogurt, along with fiber, vitamins, and antioxidants from the spinach and banana, making it an excellent choice for menopausal women following the Galveston Diet.

32. Baked sweet potato with black beans and salsa

Ingredients:
- 2 medium sweet potatoes
- 1 can (15 ounces) black beans, drained and rinsed
- 1 cup salsa (homemade or store-bought)
- 1 avocado, diced
- Fresh cilantro, chopped (for garnish, optional)
- Lime wedges (for serving, optional)

Instructions:

1. Preheat your oven to 400°F (200°C).

2. Wash the sweet potatoes and pierce them several times with a fork. Place them on a baking sheet lined with parchment paper or aluminum foil.

3. Bake the sweet potatoes in the preheated oven for 45-60 minutes, or until they are tender and easily pierced with a fork.

4. While the sweet potatoes are baking, prepare the black beans: In a small saucepan, heat the black beans over medium heat until warmed through. You can season them with a pinch of salt and pepper if desired.

5. Once the sweet potatoes are done baking, remove them from the oven and let them cool slightly.

6. To serve, slice each sweet potato open lengthwise and fluff the flesh with a fork. Top each sweet potato with a portion of warm black beans, followed by a spoonful of salsa.

7. Garnish the baked sweet potatoes with diced avocado and chopped fresh cilantro, if desired.

8. Serve the baked sweet potatoes with black beans and salsa immediately, with lime wedges on the side for squeezing over the toppings if desired.

Enjoy this flavorful and nutritious Baked Sweet Potato with Black Beans and Salsa as a satisfying meal that's perfect for supporting overall health during menopause.

This recipe provides complex carbohydrates, fiber, plant-based protein, vitamins, and minerals from the sweet potatoes, black beans, salsa, and avocado, making it an excellent choice for menopausal women following the Galveston Diet.

33. Quinoa and vegetable stir-fry

Ingredients:

- 1 cup quinoa, rinsed
- 2 cups water or vegetable broth
- 2 tablespoons olive oil
- 2 cloves garlic, minced
- 1 onion, diced
- 2 carrots, diced
- 1 bell pepper, diced
- 1 zucchini, diced
- 1 cup broccoli florets
- 1 cup snap peas, trimmed
- 1/4 cup soy sauce or tamari
- 1 tablespoon rice vinegar
- 1 tablespoon honey or maple syrup
- 1 teaspoon grated ginger
- 1 tablespoon sesame oil
- Salt and pepper to taste
- Optional garnish: sliced green onions, sesame seeds

Instructions:

1. In a medium saucepan, combine the quinoa and water or vegetable broth. Bring to a boil, then reduce the heat to low, cover, and simmer for 15-20 minutes, or until the quinoa is cooked and the liquid is absorbed. Remove from heat and set aside.

2. In a large skillet or wok, heat the olive oil over medium-high heat. Add the minced garlic and diced onion to the skillet. Cook for 2-3 minutes, or until the onion is translucent and fragrant.

3. Add the diced carrots, bell pepper, zucchini, broccoli florets, and snap peas to the skillet. Stir-fry for 5-7 minutes, or until the vegetables are tender-crisp.

4. In a small bowl, whisk together the soy sauce or tamari, rice vinegar, honey or maple syrup, grated ginger, and sesame oil to make the sauce.

5. Pour the sauce over the stir-fried vegetables in the skillet. Stir well to coat the vegetables evenly with the sauce.

6. Add the cooked quinoa to the skillet with the vegetables and sauce. Stir well to combine. Cook for an additional 2-3 minutes, or until everything is heated through.

7. Taste the stir-fry and adjust the seasoning with salt and pepper if needed. Once everything is heated through and well combined, remove the skillet from the heat.

8. Serve the quinoa and vegetable stir-fry hot, garnished with sliced green onions and sesame seeds if desired.

Enjoy this flavorful and nutritious Quinoa and Vegetable Stir-Fry as a satisfying meal that's perfect for supporting overall health during menopause.

This recipe provides complex carbohydrates, plant-based protein, fiber, vitamins, and minerals from the quinoa and an assortment of colorful vegetables, making it an excellent choice for menopausal women following the Galveston Diet. Enjoy!

34. Salmon salad with mixed greens

Ingredients:
For the Salmon:
- 2 salmon fillets
(about 6 ounces each), skin removed
- 1 tablespoon olive oil
- Salt and pepper to taste
- Lemon wedges for serving

For the Dressing:
- 2 tablespoons extra virgin olive oil
- 1 tablespoon balsamic vinegar
- 1 teaspoon Dijon mustard, 1 teaspoon honey or maple syrup, Salt and pepper to taste

For the Salad:
- 4 cups mixed salad greens (such as spinach, arugula, and kale)
- 1 cucumber, sliced
- 1 cup cherry tomatoes, halved
- 1/4 red onion, thinly sliced
- 1/4 cup Kalamata olives, pitted
- Optional add-ins: sliced avocado, crumbled feta cheese, toasted nuts or seeds

Instructions:

1. Preheat your grill or grill pan over medium-high heat.

2. Pat the salmon fillets dry with paper towels. Brush both sides of each fillet with olive oil and season with salt and pepper.

3. Place the salmon fillets on the preheated grill or grill pan and cook for 3-4 minutes per side, or until the salmon is cooked through and flakes easily with a fork. Remove from heat and set aside.

4. While the salmon is cooking, prepare the salad ingredients: In a large salad bowl, combine the mixed greens, sliced cucumber, cherry tomatoes, thinly sliced red onion, and Kalamata olives. Add any optional add-ins such as sliced avocado, crumbled feta cheese, or toasted nuts or seeds if desired.

5. In a small bowl, whisk together the extra virgin olive oil, balsamic vinegar, Dijon mustard, honey or maple syrup, salt, and pepper to make the dressing.

6. Once the salmon is cooked, flake it into large chunks with a fork. Add the flaked salmon to the salad bowl with the mixed greens and vegetables.

7. Drizzle the dressing over the salad and toss gently to coat everything evenly with the dressing. Divide the salmon salad among serving plates.

8. Serve the salmon salad immediately, garnished with lemon wedges for squeezing over the salmon if desired.

Enjoy this delicious and nutritious Salmon Salad with Mixed Greens as a satisfying meal that's perfect for supporting overall health during menopause. This recipe provides omega-3 fatty acids, protein, fiber, vitamins, and minerals from the salmon and mixed greens, making it an excellent choice for menopausal women following the Galveston Diet.

35. Turkey chili with quinoa

Ingredients:

- 1 tablespoon olive oil
- 1 onion, diced
- 2 cloves garlic, minced
- 1 bell pepper, diced
- 2 carrots, diced
- 1 zucchini, diced
- 1 lb ground turkey
- 1 can (14 ounces) diced tomatoes
- 1/2 cup quinoa, rinsed
- 2 tablespoons chili powder
- 1 can (15 ounces) black beans, drained and rinsed
- 4 cups vegetable broth or chicken broth
- 1 teaspoon ground cumin
- 1 teaspoon paprika
- 1/2 teaspoon dried oregano
- 1 can (15 ounces) kidney beans, drained and rinsed
- Salt and pepper to taste
- Optional toppings: shredded cheese, sliced green onions, chopped cilantro, avocado slices, Greek yogurt or sour cream

Instructions:

1. Heat the olive oil in a large pot or Dutch oven over medium heat. Add the diced onion and minced garlic to the pot. Cook for 2-3 minutes, or until the onion is translucent and fragrant.

2. Add the diced bell pepper, carrots, and zucchini to the pot. Cook for 5-7 minutes, or until the vegetables are tender.

3. Push the vegetables to one side of the pot and add the ground turkey to the empty space. Cook, breaking up the turkey with a spoon, until it is browned and cooked through.

4. Once the turkey is cooked, stir it into the cooked vegetables in the pot.

5. Add the diced tomatoes (with their juices), drained and rinsed kidney beans, drained and rinsed black beans, vegetable broth or chicken broth, rinsed quinoa, chili powder, ground cumin, paprika, dried oregano, salt, and pepper to the pot. Stir well to combine.

6. Bring the chili to a simmer, then reduce the heat to low. Cover and let the chili simmer gently for 20-25 minutes, or until the quinoa is cooked and the flavors have melded together.

7. Taste the chili and adjust the seasoning with more salt and pepper if needed. Once the chili is done cooking, remove it from the heat.

8. Serve the turkey chili hot, garnished with your choice of toppings such as shredded cheese, sliced green onions, chopped cilantro, avocado slices, or Greek yogurt/sour cream.

Enjoy this flavorful and nutritious Turkey Chili with Quinoa as a satisfying meal that's perfect for supporting overall health during menopause. This recipe provides lean protein, fiber, complex carbohydrates, vitamins, and minerals from the turkey, quinoa, beans, and assortment of vegetables, making it an excellent choice for menopausal women following the Galveston Diet.

36. Veggie wrap with hummus

Ingredients:
- 1 large whole grain or gluten-free tortilla wrap
- 2 tablespoons hummus (store-bought or homemade)
- 1/4 cup shredded carrots
- 1/4 cup sliced cucumber
- 1/4 cup sliced bell peppers (any color)
- 1/4 cup baby spinach or mixed greens
- 1/4 avocado, sliced
- Optional add-ins: sliced tomatoes, shredded cabbage, sprouts, shredded beets
- Optional seasonings: salt, pepper, dried herbs, red pepper flakes

Instructions:

1. Lay the tortilla wrap flat on a clean surface.

2. Spread the hummus evenly over the surface of the tortilla, leaving a small border around the edges.

3. Layer the shredded carrots, sliced cucumber, sliced bell peppers, baby spinach or mixed greens, and sliced avocado over the hummus in the center of the tortilla.

4. Add any optional add-ins such as sliced tomatoes, shredded cabbage, sprouts, or shredded beets if desired.

5. Optionally, sprinkle the veggies with a pinch of salt, pepper, dried herbs, or red pepper flakes for extra flavor.

6. Fold in the sides of the tortilla, then roll it up tightly from the bottom to enclose the filling, creating a wrap.

7. Slice the veggie wrap in half diagonally or into smaller pinwheels, if desired.

8. Serve the veggie wrap immediately, or wrap it tightly in foil or parchment paper for later enjoyment.

Enjoy this delicious and nutritious Veggie Wrap with Hummus as a satisfying meal that's perfect for supporting overall health during menopause.

This recipe provides fiber, vitamins, minerals, and healthy fats from the whole grain tortilla, hummus, and assortment of colorful vegetables, making it an excellent choice for menopausal women following the Galveston Diet. Enjoy!

37. Eggplant stir-fry with tofu

Ingredients:
- 1 medium eggplant, cubed
- 1 block (14-16 ounces) firm tofu, drained and cubed
- 2 tablespoons soy sauce or tamari
- 2 tablespoons rice vinegar
- 1 tablespoon honey or maple syrup
- 1 tablespoon sesame oil
- 2 cloves garlic, minced
- 1 teaspoon grated ginger
- 2 tablespoons olive oil or vegetable oil
- 1 bell pepper, sliced
- 1 onion, sliced
- 2 cups broccoli florets
- Salt and pepper to taste
- Cooked brown rice or quinoa for serving
- Optional garnish: sliced green onions, sesame seeds

Instructions:

1. In a small bowl, whisk together the soy sauce or tamari, rice vinegar, honey or maple syrup, sesame oil, minced garlic, and grated ginger to make the stir-fry sauce. Set aside.

2. Heat one tablespoon of olive oil or vegetable oil in a large skillet or wok over medium-high heat. Add the cubed tofu to the skillet and cook for 5-7 minutes, or until golden brown and crispy on all sides. Remove the tofu from the skillet and set aside.

3. In the same skillet, add another tablespoon of olive oil or vegetable oil if needed. Add the cubed eggplant to the skillet and cook for 5-7 minutes, or until the eggplant is softened and lightly browned.

4. Add the sliced bell pepper, sliced onion, and broccoli florets to the skillet with the eggplant. Stir-fry for an additional 4-5 minutes, or until the vegetables are tender-crisp.

5. Return the cooked tofu to the skillet with the vegetables.

6. Pour the prepared stir-fry sauce over the tofu and vegetables in the skillet. Stir well to coat everything evenly with the sauce.

7. Cook for an additional 2-3 minutes, or until the sauce has thickened slightly and everything is heated through.

8. Taste the stir-fry and adjust the seasoning with salt and pepper if needed. Once everything is heated through and well combined, remove the skillet from the heat.

10. Serve the eggplant stir-fry with tofu immediately over cooked brown rice or quinoa. Garnish with sliced green onions and sesame seeds if desired.

Enjoy this flavorful and nutritious Eggplant Stir-Fry with Tofu as a satisfying meal that's perfect for supporting overall health during menopause.

This recipe provides plant-based protein, fiber, vitamins, and minerals from the tofu, eggplant, and assortment of colorful vegetables, making it an excellent choice for menopausal women following the Galveston Diet.

38. Grilled shrimp with quinoa salad

Ingredients:

For the Grilled Shrimp:
- 1 lb large shrimp, peeled and deveined
- 2 tablespoons olive oil
- 2 cloves garlic, minced
- 1 teaspoon smoked paprika
- Salt and pepper to taste
- Lemon wedges for serving

For the Quinoa Salad:
- 1 cup quinoa, rinsed
- 2 cups water or vegetable broth
- 1 cucumber, diced
- 1 bell pepper, diced
- 1 cup cherry tomatoes, halved
- 1/4 red onion, thinly sliced
- 1/4 cup chopped fresh parsley or cilantro
- 2 tablespoons extra virgin olive oil
- 2 tablespoons lemon juice
- 1 teaspoon Dijon mustard
- Salt and pepper to taste

Instructions:

1. Preheat your grill to medium-high heat.

2. In a mixing bowl, combine the olive oil, minced garlic, smoked paprika, salt, and pepper. Add the peeled and deveined shrimp to the bowl and toss to coat the shrimp evenly with the marinade.

3. Thread the marinated shrimp onto skewers, if using.

4. Place the shrimp skewers on the preheated grill and cook for 2-3 minutes per side, or until the shrimp are pink and opaque. Remove from the grill and set aside.

5. In a medium saucepan, combine the quinoa and water or vegetable broth. Bring to a boil, then reduce the heat to low, cover, and simmer for 15-20 minutes, or until the quinoa is cooked and the liquid is absorbed. Remove from heat and let it cool slightly.

6. In a large salad bowl, combine the cooked quinoa, diced cucumber, diced bell pepper, halved cherry tomatoes, thinly sliced red onion, and chopped fresh parsley or cilantro.

7. In a small bowl, whisk together the extra virgin olive oil, lemon juice, Dijon mustard, salt, and pepper to make the dressing.

8. Pour the dressing over the quinoa salad and toss well to coat everything evenly. Serve the grilled shrimp skewers alongside the quinoa salad.

10. Garnish the quinoa salad with additional chopped fresh parsley or cilantro if desired. Serve with lemon wedges for squeezing over the grilled shrimp, if desired.

Enjoy this delicious and nutritious Grilled Shrimp with Quinoa Salad as a satisfying meal that's perfect for supporting overall health during menopause.

This recipe provides lean protein, fiber, complex carbohydrates, vitamins, and minerals from the shrimp, quinoa, and assortment of colorful vegetables, making it an excellent choice for menopausal women following the Galveston Diet. Enjoy!

39. Greek yogurt with honey and walnuts

Ingredients:
- 1 cup Greek yogurt (low-fat or full-fat, according to preference)
- 1-2 tablespoons honey (adjust to taste)
- 2 tablespoons chopped walnuts
- Optional: fresh berries or sliced fruit for garnish

Instructions:

1. Spoon the Greek yogurt into a serving bowl.

2. Drizzle the honey over the Greek yogurt. Sprinkle the chopped walnuts on top of the yogurt and honey.

3. If desired, garnish with fresh berries or sliced fruit. Serve immediately and enjoy!

This simple and nutritious Greek Yogurt with Honey and Walnuts makes a delicious breakfast, snack, or dessert option that's perfect for supporting overall health during menopause.

Greek yogurt provides protein, probiotics, and calcium, while honey adds natural sweetness and walnuts contribute healthy fats and crunch. This combination is rich in nutrients and can help satisfy hunger and cravings while providing essential nutrients for menopausal women following the Galveston Diet.

40. Lentil and vegetable stew

Ingredients:
- 1 cup dried lentils, rinsed and drained
- 4 cups vegetable broth
- 2 tablespoons olive oil
- 1 onion, diced
- 2 carrots, diced
- 2 celery stalks, diced
- 2 cloves garlic, minced
- 1 bell pepper, diced
- 1 zucchini, diced
- 1 can (14 ounces) diced tomatoes
- 1 teaspoon dried thyme
- 1 teaspoon dried oregano
- 1 teaspoon smoked paprika
- Salt and pepper to taste
- 2 cups chopped spinach or kale
- Optional garnish: chopped fresh parsley or cilantro

Instructions:

1. In a large pot or Dutch oven, heat the olive oil over medium heat. Add the diced onion, carrots, and celery to the pot. Cook for 5-7 minutes, or until the vegetables are softened.

2. Add the minced garlic to the pot and cook for an additional minute, or until fragrant.

3. Stir in the diced bell pepper, diced zucchini, dried thyme, dried oregano, and smoked paprika. Cook for another 2-3 minutes.

4. Add the rinsed lentils, vegetable broth, and diced tomatoes (with their juices) to the pot. Stir well to combine.

5. Bring the stew to a simmer, then reduce the heat to low. Cover and let the stew simmer gently for 25-30 minutes, or until the lentils are tender.

6. Once the lentils are tender, stir in the chopped spinach or kale. Cook for an additional 2-3 minutes, or until the greens are wilted.

7. Taste the stew and adjust the seasoning with salt and pepper as needed. Remove the pot from the heat.

9. Serve the lentil and vegetable stew hot, garnished with chopped fresh parsley or cilantro if desired.

Enjoy this hearty and nutritious Lentil and Vegetable Stew as a satisfying meal that's perfect for supporting overall health during menopause.

This recipe provides plant-based protein, fiber, vitamins, and minerals from the lentils and assortment of colorful vegetables, making it an excellent choice for menopausal women following the Galveston Diet.

41. Roasted chicken with cauliflower rice

Ingredients:
For the Roasted Chicken:
- 4 bone-in, skin-on chicken thighs or breasts
- 2 tablespoons olive oil
- 2 cloves garlic, minced
- 1 teaspoon dried thyme
- 1 teaspoon dried rosemary
- Salt and pepper to taste

For the Cauliflower Rice:
- 1 head cauliflower, cut into florets
- 2 tablespoons olive oil
- 2 cloves garlic, minced
- Salt and pepper to taste
- Optional: chopped fresh parsley for garnish

Instructions:
1. Preheat your oven to 400°F (200°C).

2. Place the chicken thighs or breasts on a baking sheet lined with parchment paper or aluminum foil.

3. In a small bowl, mix together the olive oil, minced garlic, dried thyme, dried rosemary, salt, and pepper. Brush or rub the mixture evenly over the chicken pieces.

4. Roast the chicken in the preheated oven for 25-30 minutes, or until the chicken is cooked through and reaches an internal temperature of 165°F (74°C). If using bone-in, skin-on chicken thighs, they may need a few extra minutes to cook through.

5. While the chicken is roasting, prepare the cauliflower rice. Place the cauliflower florets in a food processor and pulse until they resemble rice-like grains.

6. Heat the olive oil in a large skillet over medium heat. Add the minced garlic to the skillet and cook for 1-2 minutes, or until fragrant.

7. Add the riced cauliflower to the skillet and cook for 5-7 minutes, stirring occasionally, until the cauliflower is tender.

8. Season the cauliflower rice with salt and pepper to taste.

9. Once the chicken is done roasting and the cauliflower rice is cooked, remove them from the oven and skillet, respectively.

10. Serve the roasted chicken alongside the cauliflower rice. Garnish with chopped fresh parsley, if desired.

Enjoy this delicious and nutritious Roasted Chicken with Cauliflower Rice as a satisfying meal that's perfect for supporting overall health during menopause.

This recipe provides lean protein, fiber, vitamins, and minerals from the chicken and cauliflower, making it an excellent choice for menopausal women following the Galveston Diet.

42. Bean salad with bell peppers and corn

Ingredients:
- 1 can (15 ounces) black beans, drained and rinsed
- 1 can (15 ounces) kidney beans, drained and rinsed
- 1 cup corn kernels (fresh, frozen, or canned)
- 1 red bell pepper, diced
- 1 yellow bell pepper, diced
- 1/2 red onion, diced
- 2 tablespoons lime juice
- 1 teaspoon ground cumin
- 1/4 cup chopped fresh cilantro
- 2 tablespoons extra virgin olive oil
- 1/2 teaspoon chili powder
- Salt and pepper to taste
- Optional add-ins: diced avocado, cherry tomatoes, diced cucumber

Instructions:

1. In a large salad bowl, combine the black beans, kidney beans, corn kernels, diced red bell pepper, diced yellow bell pepper, diced red onion, and chopped fresh cilantro.

2. In a small bowl, whisk together the extra virgin olive oil, lime juice, ground cumin, chili powder, salt, and pepper to make the dressing.

3. Pour the dressing over the bean salad in the bowl. Toss well to coat everything evenly with the dressing.

4. Taste the bean salad and adjust the seasoning with more salt and pepper if needed.

5. If desired, add any optional add-ins such as diced avocado, cherry tomatoes, or diced cucumber to the salad and toss gently to combine.

6. Once everything is well combined and seasoned to your liking, cover the salad bowl and refrigerate for at least 30 minutes to allow the flavors to meld together.

7. Before serving, give the bean salad a final toss to redistribute the dressing. Serve the bean salad chilled as a side dish or light meal.

Enjoy this delicious and nutritious Bean Salad with Bell Peppers and Corn as a satisfying meal that's perfect for supporting overall health during menopause.

This recipe provides fiber, plant-based protein, vitamins, and minerals from the beans, bell peppers, corn, and assortment of colorful vegetables, making it an excellent choice for menopausal women following the Galveston Diet.

43. Veggie omelet with whole grain toast

Ingredients:

For the Veggie Omelet:
- 2 large eggs
- 1/4 cup diced bell peppers (any color)
- 1/4 cup diced tomatoes
- 1/4 cup diced onion
- 1/4 cup chopped spinach or kale
- Salt and pepper to taste
- 1 tablespoon olive oil or cooking spray
- Optional add-ins: diced mushrooms, diced zucchini, shredded cheese

For the Whole Grain Toast:
- 2 slices whole grain bread
- Butter or avocado for spreading (optional)

Instructions:

1. In a small bowl, whisk together the eggs until well beaten. Season with salt and pepper to taste.

2. Heat the olive oil or cooking spray in a non-stick skillet over medium heat.

3. Add the diced bell peppers, diced tomatoes, diced onion, and chopped spinach or kale to the skillet. Cook for 2-3 minutes, or until the vegetables are softened.

4. Pour the beaten eggs over the cooked vegetables in the skillet. Tilt the skillet to spread the eggs evenly over the vegetables.

5. Allow the omelet to cook undisturbed for 2-3 minutes, or until the edges are set and the bottom is lightly golden brown.

6. Using a spatula, carefully fold one side of the omelet over the other to create a half-moon shape. Cook for another 1-2 minutes, or until the eggs are cooked through.

7. Slide the veggie omelet onto a plate and set aside. Toast the whole grain bread slices until golden brown.

8. Spread butter or avocado on the toasted bread slices, if desired. Serve the veggie omelet hot with whole grain toast on the side.

9. Optionally, garnish the omelet with chopped fresh herbs or shredded cheese before serving.

Enjoy this delicious and nutritious Veggie Omelet with Whole Grain Toast as a satisfying breakfast or brunch option that's perfect for supporting overall health during menopause.

This recipe provides protein, fiber, vitamins, and minerals from the eggs, vegetables, and whole grain bread, making it an excellent choice for menopausal women following the Galveston Diet.

44. Black bean soup with avocado

Ingredients:
- 2 cans (15 ounces each) black beans, drained and rinsed
- 1 tablespoon olive oil
- 1 onion, diced
- 2 cloves garlic, minced
- 1 bell pepper, diced
- 2 carrots, diced
- 2 stalks celery, diced
- 1 teaspoon ground cumin
- 1 teaspoon chili powder
- 1/2 teaspoon smoked paprika
- 4 cups vegetable broth
- Salt and pepper to taste
- 1 avocado, diced
- Fresh cilantro, chopped, for garnish
- Lime wedges, for serving

Instructions:

1. Heat the olive oil in a large pot or Dutch oven over medium heat. Add the diced onion, minced garlic, diced bell pepper, diced carrots, and diced celery to the pot. Cook for 5-7 minutes, or until the vegetables are softened.

2. Stir in the ground cumin, chili powder, and smoked paprika. Cook for another 1-2 minutes, or until fragrant.

3. Add the drained and rinsed black beans to the pot, along with the vegetable broth. Stir well to combine.

4. Bring the soup to a simmer, then reduce the heat to low. Cover and let the soup simmer gently for 15-20 minutes to allow the flavors to meld together.

5. Once the soup is done simmering, use an immersion blender to blend part of the soup until creamy, leaving some beans and vegetables whole for texture. Alternatively, transfer a portion of the soup to a blender and blend until smooth, then return it to the pot.

6. Taste the soup and adjust the seasoning with salt and pepper as needed.

7. Ladle the black bean soup into serving bowls. Top each bowl with diced avocado and chopped fresh cilantro.

8. Serve the black bean soup hot, with lime wedges on the side for squeezing over the soup before eating.

Enjoy this delicious and nutritious Black Bean Soup with Avocado as a satisfying meal that's perfect for supporting overall health during menopause.

This recipe provides fiber, plant-based protein, vitamins, and minerals from the black beans, vegetables, and avocado, making it an excellent choice for menopausal women following the Galveston Diet.

45. Baked tofu with broccoli and brown rice

Ingredients:
For the Baked Tofu:
- 1 block (14-16 ounces) extra firm tofu
- 2 tablespoons soy sauce or tamari
- 1 tablespoon olive oil
- 1 tablespoon maple syrup or honey
- 1 teaspoon sesame oil
- 1 teaspoon grated ginger
- 2 cloves garlic, minced
- Optional: pinch of red pepper flakes for heat

For the Broccoli:
- 2 cups broccoli florets
- 1 tablespoon olive oil
- Salt and pepper to taste

For Serving:
- 2 cups cooked brown rice

Instructions:
1. Preheat your oven to 400°F (200°C).

2. Press the tofu: Remove the tofu from the packaging and drain any excess liquid. Wrap the tofu block in a clean kitchen towel or paper towels and place it on a plate. Place a heavy object on top of the tofu, such as a cast-iron skillet or a stack of heavy books, and let it press for 20-30 minutes to remove excess moisture.

3. While the tofu is pressing, prepare the marinade: In a small bowl, whisk together the soy sauce or tamari, olive oil, maple syrup or honey, sesame oil, grated ginger, minced garlic, and optional red pepper flakes.

4. Cut the pressed tofu into cubes or triangles and place them in a shallow dish or a large resealable plastic bag. Pour the marinade over the tofu, making sure it's evenly coated. Allow the tofu to marinate for at least 15-20 minutes, or longer if time allows.

5. While the tofu is marinating, toss the broccoli florets with olive oil, salt, and pepper in a separate bowl until evenly coated.

6. Spread the marinated tofu cubes in a single layer on a baking sheet lined with parchment paper or aluminum foil. Bake in the preheated oven for 25-30 minutes, flipping halfway through, until the tofu is golden brown and crispy on the edges.

7. During the last 15 minutes of baking time for the tofu, add the seasoned broccoli florets to the baking sheet. Roast them alongside the tofu until they are tender and lightly browned.

8. While the tofu and broccoli are baking, cook the brown rice according to package instructions.

9. Once the tofu, broccoli, and brown rice are cooked, divide them evenly among serving plates. Serve the baked tofu and broccoli alongside the brown rice.

Enjoy this delicious and nutritious Baked Tofu with Broccoli and Brown Rice as a satisfying meal that's perfect for supporting overall health during menopause.

This recipe provides plant-based protein, fiber, vitamins, and minerals from the tofu, broccoli, and brown rice, making it an excellent choice for menopausal women following the Galveston Diet.

46. Quinoa tabbouleh with cucumber and tomato

Ingredients:
- 1 cup quinoa, rinsed
- 2 cups water or vegetable broth
- 1 cucumber, diced
- 2 tomatoes, diced
- 1/2 red onion, finely chopped
- 2 tablespoons chopped fresh mint
- 1/4 cup extra virgin olive oil
- 1/4 cup chopped fresh parsley
- 1/4 cup fresh lemon juice
- 2 cloves garlic, minced
- Salt and pepper to taste

Instructions:
1. In a medium saucepan, combine the quinoa and water or vegetable broth. Bring to a boil, then reduce the heat to low, cover, and simmer for 15-20 minutes, or until the quinoa is cooked and the liquid is absorbed. Remove from heat and let it cool slightly.

2. In a large mixing bowl, combine the cooked quinoa, diced cucumber, diced tomatoes, finely chopped red onion, chopped fresh parsley, and chopped fresh mint.

3. In a small bowl, whisk together the extra virgin olive oil, fresh lemon juice, minced garlic, salt, and pepper to make the dressing.

4. Pour the dressing over the quinoa tabbouleh salad in the mixing bowl. Toss well to coat everything evenly with the dressing.

5. Taste the tabbouleh salad and adjust the seasoning with more salt and pepper if needed.

6. Once everything is well combined and seasoned to your liking, cover the bowl and refrigerate for at least 30 minutes to allow the flavors to meld together.

7. Before serving, give the quinoa tabbouleh salad a final toss to redistribute the dressing. Serve the quinoa tabbouleh chilled as a side dish or light meal.

Enjoy this delicious and nutritious Quinoa Tabbouleh with Cucumber and Tomato as a satisfying dish that's perfect for supporting overall health during menopause.

This recipe provides protein, fiber, vitamins, and minerals from the quinoa, cucumber, tomatoes, and assortment of fresh herbs, making it an excellent choice for menopausal women following the Galveston Diet.

47. Turkey and vegetable soup

Ingredients:
- 1 tablespoon olive oil
- 1 onion, diced
- 2 carrots, diced
- 2 celery stalks, diced
- 2 cloves garlic, minced
- 1 pound lean ground turkey
- 6 cups low-sodium chicken or vegetable broth
- 1 can (14 ounces) diced tomatoes
- 1 cup frozen corn kernels
- 1 cup frozen peas
- 1 teaspoon dried thyme
- 1 teaspoon dried rosemary
- Salt and pepper to taste
- Fresh parsley or cilantro, chopped, for garnish (optional)

Instructions:
1. Heat the olive oil in a large pot or Dutch oven over medium heat. Add the diced onion, carrots, and celery to the pot. Cook for 5-7 minutes, or until the vegetables are softened.

2. Add the minced garlic to the pot and cook for an additional minute, or until fragrant.

3. Add the ground turkey to the pot, breaking it up with a spoon, and cook until browned and cooked through.

4. Stir in the low-sodium chicken or vegetable broth, diced tomatoes (with their juices), frozen corn kernels, frozen peas, dried thyme, and dried rosemary. Bring the soup to a simmer.

5. Once the soup is simmering, reduce the heat to low and let it simmer gently for 20-25 minutes to allow the flavors to meld together.

6. Taste the soup and season with salt and pepper to taste. Ladle the turkey and vegetable soup into serving bowls.

8. Garnish each bowl with chopped fresh parsley or cilantro, if desired. Serve the soup hot and enjoy!

Enjoy this delicious and nutritious Turkey and Vegetable Soup as a satisfying meal that's perfect for supporting overall health during menopause.

This recipe provides lean protein, fiber, vitamins, and minerals from the ground turkey and assortment of vegetables, making it an excellent choice for menopausal women following the Galveston Diet.

48. Greek yogurt with mixed berries

Ingredients:
- 1 cup Greek yogurt (low-fat or full-fat, according to preference)
- 1/2 cup mixed berries (such as strawberries, blueberries, raspberries, blackberries)
- 1 tablespoon honey or maple syrup (optional, for added sweetness)
- Optional toppings: sliced almonds, chopped walnuts, shredded coconut

Instructions:
1. Spoon the Greek yogurt into a serving bowl or glass.

2. Wash the mixed berries and pat them dry with a paper towel. If using strawberries, remove the stems and slice them into smaller pieces.

3. Arrange the mixed berries on top of the Greek yogurt.

4. If desired, drizzle honey or maple syrup over the berries for added sweetness.

5. Optional: sprinkle sliced almonds, chopped walnuts, or shredded coconut on top for added texture and flavor.

6. Serve the Greek yogurt with mixed berries immediately and enjoy!

This Greek Yogurt with Mixed Berries is not only delicious but also packed with nutrients. Greek yogurt provides protein, probiotics, and calcium, while mixed berries offer vitamins, antioxidants, and fiber. It's a perfect snack or breakfast option for menopausal women following the Galveston Diet.

49. Stir-fried tempeh with mixed vegetables

Ingredients:
- 1 block (8 ounces) tempeh, cut into cubes or strips
- 2 tablespoons soy sauce or tamari
- 1 tablespoon rice vinegar
- 1 tablespoon maple syrup or honey
- 1 teaspoon sesame oil
- 1 teaspoon grated ginger
- 2 tablespoons olive oil or coconut oil
- 2 cups mixed vegetables (such as bell peppers, broccoli, carrots, snap peas)
- Salt and pepper to taste
- Optional garnish: sliced green onions, sesame seeds

Instructions:

1. In a small bowl, whisk together the soy sauce or tamari, rice vinegar, maple syrup or honey, sesame oil, minced garlic, and grated ginger to make the marinade.

2. Place the tempeh cubes or strips in a shallow dish and pour the marinade over them. Toss to coat the tempeh evenly with the marinade. Let it marinate for at least 15-20 minutes, or longer if time allows.

3. Heat one tablespoon of olive oil or coconut oil in a large skillet or wok over medium-high heat.

4. Add the marinated tempeh to the skillet in a single layer. Cook for 3-4 minutes, stirring occasionally, until the tempeh is browned and crispy on the edges. Remove the tempeh from the skillet and set aside.

5. In the same skillet, heat the remaining tablespoon of olive oil or coconut oil over medium-high heat.

6. Add the mixed vegetables to the skillet. Stir-fry for 4-5 minutes, or until the vegetables are tender-crisp.

7. Return the cooked tempeh to the skillet with the vegetables. Stir well to combine. Cook for an additional 1-2 minutes to heat everything through.

8. Taste the stir-fry and adjust the seasoning with salt and pepper if needed. Once everything is heated through and well combined, remove the skillet from the heat.

9. Serve the stir-fried tempeh and mixed vegetables immediately, garnished with sliced green onions and sesame seeds if desired.

Enjoy this flavorful and nutritious Stir-Fried Tempeh with Mixed Vegetables as a satisfying meal that's perfect for supporting overall health during menopause.

This recipe provides plant-based protein, fiber, vitamins, and minerals from the tempeh and assortment of colorful vegetables, making it an excellent choice for menopausal women following the Galveston Diet. Enjoy!

50. Grilled tilapia with mango salsa

Ingredients:

For the Grilled Tilapia:
- 4 tilapia fillets
- 2 tablespoons olive oil
- 1 teaspoon ground cumin
- 1 teaspoon chili powder
- Salt and pepper to taste
- Lemon wedges for serving

For the Mango Salsa:
- 1 ripe mango, peeled and diced
- 1/2 red bell pepper, diced
- 1/4 cup red onion, finely chopped
- 1 jalapeño pepper, seeded and finely chopped
- 2 tablespoons fresh cilantro, chopped
- 1 tablespoon lime juice
- Salt and pepper to taste

Instructions:

1. Preheat your grill to medium-high heat.

2. In a small bowl, mix together the olive oil, ground cumin, chili powder, salt, and pepper.

3. Brush both sides of the tilapia fillets with the seasoned olive oil mixture.

4. Place the tilapia fillets on the preheated grill and cook for 3-4 minutes per side, or until the fish is opaque and easily flakes with a fork. Cooking time may vary depending on the thickness of the fillets.

5. While the tilapia is grilling, prepare the mango salsa. In a medium bowl, combine the diced mango, diced red bell pepper, finely chopped red onion, finely chopped jalapeño pepper, chopped fresh cilantro, and lime juice. Season with salt and pepper to taste. Stir until well combined.

6. Once the tilapia fillets are cooked through, remove them from the grill and transfer to serving plates.

7. Top each grilled tilapia fillet with a generous spoonful of mango salsa.

8. Serve the grilled tilapia with mango salsa immediately, with lemon wedges on the side for squeezing over the fish if desired.

Enjoy this delicious and nutritious Grilled Tilapia with Mango Salsa as a flavorful meal that's perfect for supporting overall health during menopause.

This recipe provides lean protein, healthy fats, vitamins, and minerals from the tilapia and fresh mango salsa, making it an excellent choice for menopausal women following the Galveston Diet. Enjoy!

51. Spinach and mushroom quiche

Ingredients:
For the Quiche Crust:
- 1 1/4 cups whole wheat flour
- 1/2 teaspoon salt
- 1/2 cup cold unsalted butter, cut into small cubes
- 3-4 tablespoons ice water

For the Quiche Filling:
- 1 tablespoon olive oil
- 1 small onion, diced
- 2 cloves garlic, minced
- 8 ounces mushrooms, sliced
- 4 cups fresh spinach leaves
- 4 large eggs
- 1 cup milk (dairy or plant-based)
- 1 cup shredded cheese (such as cheddar, mozzarella, or Swiss)
- Salt and pepper to taste
- Optional: pinch of nutmeg or dried herbs (such as thyme or oregano)

Instructions:

1. Preheat your oven to 375°F (190°C).

2. In a large mixing bowl, whisk together the whole wheat flour and salt. Add the cold cubed butter to the flour mixture.

3. Use a pastry cutter or two forks to cut the butter into the flour until the mixture resembles coarse crumbs.

4. Gradually add the ice water, one tablespoon at a time, mixing with a fork, until the dough comes together and forms a ball. Be careful not to overwork the dough.

5. Transfer the dough to a lightly floured surface and roll it out into a circle large enough to fit into a 9-inch pie dish. Carefully transfer the rolled-out dough to the pie dish and press it gently into the bottom and sides. Trim any excess dough and crimp the edges as desired.

6. Prick the bottom of the pie crust with a fork to prevent air bubbles from forming during baking. Bake the crust in the preheated oven for 10-12 minutes, or until lightly golden brown. Remove from the oven and set aside.

7. While the crust is baking, prepare the quiche filling. Heat the olive oil in a large skillet over medium heat. Add the diced onion and minced garlic to the skillet and cook for 2-3 minutes, or until softened and fragrant.

8. Add the sliced mushrooms to the skillet and cook for 5-7 minutes, or until they release their moisture and become golden brown.

9. Add the fresh spinach leaves to the skillet and cook for 2-3 minutes, or until wilted. Remove the skillet from the heat and set aside.

10. In a separate mixing bowl, whisk together the eggs and milk until well combined. Season with salt, pepper, and any optional herbs or spices.

11. Spread the cooked mushroom and spinach mixture evenly over the bottom of the pre-baked pie crust. Sprinkle the shredded cheese over the top.

12. Pour the egg and milk mixture over the vegetables and cheese in the pie crust. Bake the quiche in the preheated oven for 30-35 minutes, or until the filling is set and the top is golden brown.

13. Remove the quiche from the oven and let it cool for a few minutes before slicing and serving.

Enjoy this delicious and nutritious Spinach and Mushroom Quiche as a satisfying meal that's perfect for supporting overall health during menopause.

This recipe provides protein, fiber, vitamins, and minerals from the eggs, spinach, mushrooms, and whole wheat crust, making it an excellent choice for menopausal women following the Galveston Diet.

52. Lentil salad with roasted vegetables

Ingredients:
For the Lentils:
- 1 cup dry green lentils, rinsed
- 3 cups water or vegetable broth
- 1 bay leaf
- Salt to taste

For the Roasted Vegetables:
- 2 cups mixed vegetables
(such as bell peppers, zucchini,
cherry tomatoes, red onion, carrots), diced
- 2 tablespoons olive oil

For the Dressing:
- 3 tablespoons extra virgin olive oil
- 2 tablespoons balsamic vinegar
- 1 tablespoon Dijon mustard
- 1 tablespoon maple syrup or honey
- Salt and pepper to taste

- 1 teaspoon dried thyme
- 2 cloves garlic, minced
- 1 teaspoon dried rosemary
- Salt and pepper to taste

Instructions:
1. Preheat your oven to 400°F (200°C).

2. In a medium saucepan, combine the dry green lentils, water or vegetable broth, and bay leaf. Bring to a boil over medium-high heat.

3. Reduce the heat to low, cover, and simmer for 20-25 minutes, or until the lentils are tender but still hold their shape. Drain any excess liquid and discard the bay leaf. Season the cooked lentils with salt to taste. Set aside to cool.

4. While the lentils are cooking, prepare the roasted vegetables. In a large mixing bowl, toss the diced mixed vegetables with olive oil, minced garlic, dried thyme, dried rosemary, salt, and pepper until evenly coated.

5. Spread the seasoned vegetables in a single layer on a baking sheet lined with parchment paper or aluminum foil.

6. Roast the vegetables in the preheated oven for 20-25 minutes, or until tender and lightly browned, stirring halfway through cooking.

7. While the vegetables are roasting, prepare the dressing. In a small bowl, whisk together the extra virgin olive oil, balsamic vinegar, Dijon mustard, maple syrup or honey, salt, and pepper until well combined.

8. Once the lentils are cooked and the vegetables are roasted, transfer them to a large mixing bowl. Allow them to cool slightly.

9. Pour the dressing over the lentils and roasted vegetables. Toss gently to coat everything evenly with the dressing.

10. Taste the lentil salad and adjust the seasoning with more salt and pepper if needed.

11. Serve the lentil salad with roasted vegetables at room temperature or chilled, as desired.

Enjoy this delicious and nutritious Lentil Salad with Roasted Vegetables as a satisfying meal that's perfect for supporting overall health during menopause.

This recipe provides fiber, plant-based protein, vitamins, and minerals from the lentils and assortment of colorful vegetables, making it an excellent choice for menopausal women following the Galveston Diet.

53. Chicken and vegetable curry

Ingredients:

- 1 tablespoon olive oil
- 1 onion, diced
- 2 cloves garlic, minced
- 1 tablespoon grated ginger
- 1 pound boneless, skinless chicken breasts or thighs, cut into bite-sized pieces
- 2 tablespoons curry powder
- 1 teaspoon ground turmeric
- 1 teaspoon ground cumin
- 1 teaspoon ground coriander
- 1/2 teaspoon chili powder (adjust to taste)
- 1 can (14 ounces) diced tomatoes
- 1 can (14 ounces) coconut milk
- 2 cups mixed vegetables (such as bell peppers, carrots, green beans, peas)
- Salt and pepper to taste
- Fresh cilantro, chopped, for garnish
- Cooked brown rice or quinoa, for serving

Instructions:

1. Heat the olive oil in a large skillet or Dutch oven over medium heat. Add the diced onion and cook for 3-4 minutes, or until softened.

2. Add the minced garlic and grated ginger to the skillet. Cook for an additional 1-2 minutes, or until fragrant.

3. Add the chicken pieces to the skillet and cook until browned on all sides, about 5-7 minutes.

4. Stir in the curry powder, ground turmeric, ground cumin, ground coriander, and chili powder. Cook for 1-2 minutes, stirring constantly, until the spices are fragrant.

5. Pour in the diced tomatoes (with their juices) and coconut milk. Stir well to combine. Add the mixed vegetables to the skillet. Stir to coat the vegetables in the curry sauce.

6. Bring the mixture to a simmer, then reduce the heat to low. Cover and let the curry simmer gently for 15-20 minutes, or until the chicken is cooked through and the vegetables are tender.

7. Taste the curry and season with salt and pepper as needed.

8. Once the chicken and vegetables are cooked through and the curry has thickened slightly, remove the skillet from the heat.

9. Serve the chicken and vegetable curry hot, garnished with chopped fresh cilantro, over cooked brown rice or quinoa.

Enjoy this flavorful and nutritious Chicken and Vegetable Curry as a satisfying meal that's perfect for supporting overall health during menopause.

This recipe provides protein, fiber, vitamins, and minerals from the chicken, vegetables, and aromatic spices, making it an excellent choice for menopausal women following the Galveston Diet.

54. Veggie stir-fry with tofu

Ingredients:

For the Stir-Fry:

- 2 tablespoons olive oil or sesame oil
- 1 onion, sliced
- 2 bell peppers, sliced
- 2 cups broccoli florets
- 1 cup sliced carrots
- 2 cups sliced mushrooms
- 2 cups snap peas or snow peas
- 2 cloves garlic, minced
- 1 tablespoon grated ginger
- 1/4 cup soy sauce or tamari
- 2 tablespoons rice vinegar
- 1 tablespoon maple syrup or honey
- Salt and pepper to taste
- Cooked brown rice or quinoa, for serving

For the Tofu:

- 1 block (14-16 ounces) extra firm tofu
- 2 tablespoons soy sauce or tamari
- 1 tablespoon rice vinegar
- 1 tablespoon maple syrup or honey
- 1 teaspoon sesame oil
- 2 cloves garlic, minced
- 1 teaspoon grated ginger
- 1 tablespoon cornstarch (optional, for extra crispiness)
- 2 tablespoons olive oil or sesame oil, for cooking

Instructions:

1. Start by preparing the tofu. Press the tofu to remove excess moisture. You can do this by wrapping the tofu block in a clean kitchen towel or paper towels, placing a heavy object on top (such as a cast-iron skillet), and letting it sit for about 20-30 minutes. Then, cut the pressed tofu into cubes.

2. In a bowl, whisk together soy sauce or tamari, rice vinegar, maple syrup or honey, sesame oil, minced garlic, and grated ginger. Add cornstarch if you desire extra crispiness.

3. Toss the tofu cubes in the marinade until they are evenly coated. Let them marinate for at least 15-20 minutes, or longer if time allows.

4. Heat 2 tablespoons of olive oil or sesame oil in a large skillet or wok over medium-high heat. Once hot, add the marinated tofu cubes and cook until golden brown and crispy on all sides, about 5-7 minutes. Remove tofu from the skillet and set aside.

5. In the same skillet or wok, add 2 tablespoons of olive oil or sesame oil. Add sliced onion and cook for 2-3 minutes until softened.

6. Add sliced bell peppers, broccoli florets, sliced carrots, mushrooms, and snap peas or snow peas to the skillet. Stir-fry for 5-7 minutes, or until the vegetables are tender-crisp.

7. Add minced garlic and grated ginger to the skillet, and cook for an additional 1-2 minutes until fragrant.

8. In a small bowl, whisk together soy sauce or tamari, rice vinegar, and maple syrup or honey. Pour the sauce over the vegetables in the skillet.

9. Add the cooked tofu back to the skillet and toss everything together until well coated in the sauce. Cook for another 2-3 minutes to heat everything through.

10. Season with salt and pepper to taste. Serve the veggie stir-fry with tofu hot over cooked brown rice or quinoa.

Enjoy this delicious and nutritious Veggie Stir-Fry with Tofu as a satisfying meal that's perfect for supporting overall health during menopause.

This recipe provides plant-based protein, fiber, vitamins, and minerals from the tofu and an assortment of colorful vegetables, making it an excellent choice for menopausal women following the Galveston Diet.

55. Grilled portobello mushrooms with balsamic glaze

Ingredients:
- 4 large portobello mushrooms, stems removed
- 2 tablespoons olive oil
- 2 cloves garlic, minced
- Salt and pepper to taste

Balsamic Glaze:
- 1/2 cup balsamic vinegar
- 2 tablespoons honey or maple syrup
- 1 clove garlic, minced (optional)
- Salt and pepper to taste
- Fresh parsley or basil, chopped, for garnish (optional)

Instructions:

1. Preheat your grill to medium-high heat.

2. In a small bowl, whisk together the olive oil, minced garlic, salt, and pepper. Brush both sides of the portobello mushrooms with the olive oil mixture.

3. Place the mushrooms on the preheated grill, gill-side down. Grill for 4-5 minutes, then flip and grill for an additional 4-5 minutes, or until the mushrooms are tender and slightly charred.

4. While the mushrooms are grilling, prepare the balsamic glaze. In a small saucepan, combine the balsamic vinegar, honey or maple syrup, minced garlic (if using), salt, and pepper. Bring to a simmer over medium heat.

5. Reduce the heat to low and let the glaze simmer for 8-10 minutes, or until it has thickened and reduced by half. Remove from heat and set aside.

6. Once the portobello mushrooms are grilled to your desired level of doneness, remove them from the grill and transfer to serving plates.

7. Drizzle the grilled portobello mushrooms with the balsamic glaze. Garnish with chopped fresh parsley or basil, if desired. Serve the grilled portobello mushrooms with balsamic glaze immediately.

Enjoy these delicious and nutritious Grilled Portobello Mushrooms with Balsamic Glaze as a satisfying meal that's perfect for supporting overall health during menopause.

This recipe provides fiber, vitamins, and minerals from the portobello mushrooms and the natural sweetness of the balsamic glaze, making it an excellent choice for menopausal women following the Galveston Diet.

56. Turkey and avocado wrap

Ingredients:
- 1 large whole grain or low-carb tortilla
- 4 slices of roasted turkey breast
- 1/2 avocado, sliced
- 1/4 cup shredded lettuce or spinach leaves
- 1/4 cup sliced cucumber
- 1/4 cup sliced bell pepper (any color)
- 1 tablespoon hummus or Greek yogurt (optional)
- Salt and pepper to taste

Instructions:
1. Lay the tortilla flat on a clean surface.

2. Spread the hummus or Greek yogurt (if using) evenly over the surface of the tortilla, leaving about an inch of space around the edges.

3. Place the roasted turkey breast slices on top of the hummus or Greek yogurt.

4. Arrange the sliced avocado, shredded lettuce or spinach leaves, sliced cucumber, and sliced bell pepper on top of the turkey slices.

5. Season the filling with salt and pepper to taste.

6. Fold the bottom edge of the tortilla over the filling, then fold in the sides, and roll it up tightly from the bottom to form a wrap.

7. Slice the wrap in half diagonally if desired, and serve immediately, or wrap it in parchment paper or foil for later.

8. Enjoy your Turkey and Avocado Wrap as a satisfying and nutritious meal!

This recipe provides lean protein, healthy fats, fiber, vitamins, and minerals from the turkey, avocado, and assorted vegetables, making it an excellent choice for menopausal women following the Galveston Diet.

57. Greek yogurt with sliced peaches and almonds

Ingredients:
- 1/2 cup Greek yogurt (low-fat or full-fat, according to preference)
- 1 ripe peach, sliced
- 2 tablespoons sliced almonds
- 1 teaspoon honey or maple syrup (optional, for added sweetness)
- Pinch of cinnamon (optional)

Instructions:

1. Spoon the Greek yogurt into a serving bowl or glass. Arrange the sliced peaches on top of the Greek yogurt.

2. Sprinkle the sliced almonds over the peaches.

3. If desired, drizzle honey or maple syrup over the peaches and almonds for added sweetness.

4. Optional: sprinkle a pinch of cinnamon over the top for extra flavor. Serve immediately and enjoy!

This Greek Yogurt with Sliced Peaches and Almonds is not only delicious but also packed with nutrients. Greek yogurt provides protein, probiotics, and calcium, while peaches offer vitamins, antioxidants, and fiber. Almonds add healthy fats, protein, and crunch to the dish. It's a perfect snack or breakfast option for menopausal women following the Galveston Diet.

58. Cauliflower crust pizza with vegetables

Ingredients:
For the Cauliflower Crust:
- 1 medium head of cauliflower, cut into florets
- 1/2 cup shredded mozzarella cheese
- 1/4 cup grated Parmesan cheese
- 1 teaspoon dried oregano
- 1/2 teaspoon garlic powder
- 1/4 teaspoon salt
- 2 large eggs, lightly beaten

For the Pizza Toppings:
- 1/2 cup tomato sauce or marinara sauce (no added sugar)
- 1 cup shredded mozzarella cheese
- Assorted vegetables of your choice (such as bell peppers, mushrooms, onions, spinach, cherry tomatoes)
- Fresh basil leaves, torn, for garnish (optional)
- Red pepper flakes, for garnish (optional)

Instructions:

1. Preheat your oven to 425°F (220°C). Line a baking sheet with parchment paper and set aside.

2. Place the cauliflower florets in a food processor and pulse until they resemble fine crumbs, similar to rice.

3. Transfer the cauliflower crumbs to a microwave-safe bowl and microwave on high for 5-6 minutes, or until softened. Allow the cauliflower to cool slightly.

4. Once cooled, transfer the cauliflower to a clean kitchen towel or cheesecloth. Squeeze out as much liquid as possible from the cauliflower. This step is crucial to ensure a crispy crust.

5. In a large mixing bowl, combine the squeezed cauliflower, shredded mozzarella cheese, grated Parmesan cheese, dried oregano, garlic powder, salt, and beaten eggs. Mix until well combined.

6. Transfer the cauliflower mixture to the prepared baking sheet. Use your hands to press the mixture into a thin, even layer, forming a round pizza crust shape.

7. Bake the cauliflower crust in the preheated oven for 15-20 minutes, or until golden brown and set.

8. Remove the cauliflower crust from the oven and spread the tomato sauce evenly over the surface.

9. Sprinkle shredded mozzarella cheese over the tomato sauce, then arrange your desired vegetables on top.

10. Return the pizza to the oven and bake for an additional 10-15 minutes, or until the cheese is melted and bubbly, and the crust edges are golden brown.

11. Once cooked, remove the pizza from the oven and let it cool slightly before slicing.

12. Garnish with torn fresh basil leaves and red pepper flakes, if desired.

13. Slice the cauliflower crust pizza into wedges and serve immediately.

Enjoy this delicious and nutritious Cauliflower Crust Pizza with Vegetables as a satisfying meal that's perfect for supporting overall health during menopause.

This recipe provides fiber, vitamins, and minerals from the cauliflower crust and an assortment of colorful vegetables, making it an excellent choice for menopausal women following the Galveston Diet.

59. Baked cod with lemon and herbs

Ingredients:
- 4 cod fillets (about 6 ounces each)
- 2 tablespoons olive oil
- 2 cloves garlic, minced
- Zest of 1 lemon
- Juice of 1 lemon
- 1 tablespoon chopped fresh parsley
- 1 tablespoon chopped fresh dill (or 1 teaspoon dried dill)
- Salt and pepper to taste
- Lemon slices for garnish (optional)
- Fresh herbs for garnish (optional)

Instructions:

1. Preheat your oven to 400°F (200°C). Lightly grease a baking dish with olive oil or cooking spray and set aside.

2. In a small bowl, whisk together the olive oil, minced garlic, lemon zest, lemon juice, chopped parsley, chopped dill, salt, and pepper.

3. Pat the cod fillets dry with paper towels and place them in the prepared baking dish.

4. Pour the lemon and herb mixture over the cod fillets, making sure they are evenly coated.

5. Arrange lemon slices on top of each cod fillet for extra flavor (optional).

6. Bake the cod in the preheated oven for 12-15 minutes, or until the fish is opaque and flakes easily with a fork.

7. Once cooked, remove the cod from the oven and let it rest for a few minutes before serving.

8. Garnish with fresh herbs if desired and serve hot.

Enjoy this delicious and nutritious Baked Cod with Lemon and Herbs as a satisfying meal that's perfect for supporting overall health during menopause.

This recipe provides lean protein, omega-3 fatty acids, and antioxidants from the cod, along with the refreshing flavor of lemon and aromatic herbs, making it an excellent choice for menopausal women following the Galveston Diet. Enjoy!

60. Lentil and kale salad with tahini dressing

Ingredients:
For the Salad:
- 1 cup dry green lentils
- 4 cups water or vegetable broth
- 1 bunch kale, stems removed and leaves chopped
- 1/2 cup cherry tomatoes, halved
- 1/4 cup red onion, thinly sliced
- 1/4 cup chopped fresh parsley
- 1/4 cup chopped fresh cilantro
- 1/4 cup chopped fresh mint (optional)
- 1/4 cup toasted pumpkin seeds or sunflower seeds (optional)
- Salt and pepper to taste

For the Tahini Dressing:
- 1/4 cup tahini
- 2 tablespoons lemon juice
- 2 tablespoons water
- 1 tablespoon olive oil
- 1 clove garlic, minced
- 1 teaspoon maple syrup or honey (optional)
- Salt and pepper to taste

Instructions:

1. Rinse the lentils under cold water. In a medium saucepan, combine the lentils and water or vegetable broth. Bring to a boil, then reduce the heat to low and simmer for 20-25 minutes, or until the lentils are tender but still hold their shape. Drain any excess liquid and set aside to cool.

2. In a large mixing bowl, add the chopped kale leaves. Massage the kale with your hands for a few minutes until it becomes tender and darker in color.

3. Add the cooked lentils, cherry tomatoes, red onion, chopped parsley, chopped cilantro, and chopped mint (if using) to the bowl with the kale. Toss to combine.

4. In a small bowl, whisk together the tahini, lemon juice, water, olive oil, minced garlic, maple syrup or honey (if using), salt, and pepper until smooth and creamy.

5. Pour the tahini dressing over the salad and toss until everything is well coated.

6. Taste and adjust seasoning with more salt, pepper, or lemon juice if needed.

7. Sprinkle toasted pumpkin seeds or sunflower seeds over the salad for added crunch and nutrition (if using).

8. Serve the lentil and kale salad immediately, or refrigerate for 30 minutes to allow the flavors to meld before serving.

Enjoy this delicious and nutritious Lentil and Kale Salad with Tahini Dressing as a satisfying meal that's perfect for supporting overall health during menopause.

This recipe provides fiber, plant-based protein, vitamins, minerals, and healthy fats from the lentils, kale, and tahini, making it an excellent choice for menopausal women following the Galveston Diet.

61. Chicken and vegetable kebabs with tzatziki sauce

Ingredients:
For the Chicken and Vegetable Kebabs:
- 1 pound boneless, skinless chicken breasts, cut into chunks
- 1 zucchini, cut into chunks
- 1 red bell pepper, cut into chunks
- 1 red onion, cut into chunks
- 8-10 cherry tomatoes
- Wooden or metal skewers
- 2 tablespoons olive oil
- 2 cloves garlic, minced
- 1 teaspoon dried oregano
- 1 teaspoon dried thyme
- Salt and pepper to taste

For the Tzatziki Sauce:
- 1 cup Greek yogurt
- 1/2 cucumber, grated and squeezed to remove excess moisture
- 1 clove garlic, minced
- 1 tablespoon lemon juice
- 1 tablespoon extra virgin olive oil
- 1 tablespoon chopped fresh dill
- Salt and pepper to taste

Instructions:

1. If using wooden skewers, soak them in water for at least 30 minutes to prevent them from burning on the grill.

2. In a mixing bowl, combine the olive oil, minced garlic, dried oregano, dried thyme, salt, and pepper. Add the chicken chunks to the bowl and toss to coat evenly. Let marinate for at least 30 minutes in the refrigerator.

3. While the chicken is marinating, prepare the vegetables by cutting them into chunks. Preheat your grill to medium-high heat.

4. Thread the marinated chicken chunks and prepared vegetables onto the skewers, alternating between chicken and vegetables.

5. Place the skewers on the preheated grill and cook for 10-12 minutes, turning occasionally, or until the chicken is cooked through and the vegetables are tender and slightly charred.

6. While the kebabs are cooking, prepare the tzatziki sauce. In a small bowl, combine the Greek yogurt, grated cucumber, minced garlic, lemon juice, extra virgin olive oil, chopped fresh dill, salt, and pepper. Mix well until smooth and creamy.

7. Once the kebabs are cooked, remove them from the grill and let them rest for a few minutes.

8. Serve the chicken and vegetable kebabs hot off the grill with a side of tzatziki sauce for dipping. Enjoy your delicious and nutritious Chicken and Vegetable Kebabs with Tzatziki Sauce as a satisfying meal that's perfect for supporting overall health during menopause.

This recipe provides lean protein, fiber, vitamins, minerals, and healthy fats from the chicken, vegetables, Greek yogurt, and olive oil, making it an excellent choice for menopausal women following the Galveston Diet.

62. Veggie burger lettuce wraps

Ingredients:
For the Veggie Burgers:
- 1 (15 oz) can black beans, drained and rinsed
- 1 cup cooked quinoa
- 1/2 cup finely chopped bell pepper (any color)
- 1/2 cup grated carrot
- 1/4 cup finely chopped red onion
- 2 cloves garlic, minced
- 1 teaspoon ground cumin
- 1 teaspoon smoked paprika
- 1/2 teaspoon chili powder
- Salt and pepper to taste
- 1/4 cup breadcrumbs or almond flour (optional, for binding)

For the Lettuce Wraps:
- Large lettuce leaves (such as butter lettuce or romaine)
- Sliced avocado
- Sliced tomato
- Sliced red onion
- Dijon mustard or your favorite sauce for topping

Instructions:

1. Preheat your oven to 375°F (190°C). Line a baking sheet with parchment paper and set aside.

2. In a large mixing bowl, mash the black beans with a fork or potato masher until mostly mashed but still some whole beans remain.

3. Add the cooked quinoa, chopped bell pepper, grated carrot, chopped red onion, minced garlic, ground cumin, smoked paprika, chili powder, salt, and pepper to the bowl with the mashed black beans. Mix until well combined.

4. If the mixture seems too wet, you can add breadcrumbs or almond flour to help bind the ingredients together. Start with a small amount and add more as needed until you reach a consistency that holds together well.

5. Form the veggie burger mixture into patties of your desired size and thickness. Place them on the prepared baking sheet.

6. Bake the veggie burgers in the preheated oven for 20-25 minutes, flipping halfway through cooking, or until they are firm and lightly browned on the outside.

7. While the veggie burgers are baking, prepare your lettuce wraps by washing and drying the lettuce leaves. Arrange the lettuce leaves on a serving platter.

8. Once the veggie burgers are cooked, assemble the lettuce wraps by placing a veggie burger patty on each lettuce leaf.

9. Top the veggie burger patties with sliced avocado, sliced tomato, sliced red onion, and your favorite sauce or condiments. Serve the veggie burger lettuce wraps immediately and enjoy.

63. Quinoa stuffed mushrooms

Ingredients:

- 12 large mushrooms (such as white button or cremini)
- 1 cup cooked quinoa
- 1/2 cup chopped onion
- 1/2 cup chopped bell pepper (any color)
- 2 cloves garlic, minced
- 1 tablespoon olive oil
- 1/4 cup chopped fresh parsley
- 1/4 cup grated Parmesan cheese (optional)
- Salt and pepper to taste
- Lemon wedges, for serving (optional)

Instructions:

1. Preheat your oven to 375°F (190°C). Line a baking sheet with parchment paper and set aside.

2. Clean the mushrooms by wiping them with a damp paper towel or gently rinsing them under cold water. Remove the stems from the mushrooms and chop them finely. Set aside.

3. In a skillet, heat the olive oil over medium heat. Add the chopped onion and bell pepper to the skillet and cook for 3-4 minutes, or until softened.

4. Add the minced garlic and chopped mushroom stems to the skillet and cook for an additional 2-3 minutes, until the mushrooms release their juices and the mixture is fragrant.

5. In a mixing bowl, combine the cooked quinoa, sautéed vegetable mixture, chopped parsley, and grated Parmesan cheese (if using). Season with salt and pepper to taste.

6. Fill each mushroom cap with a spoonful of the quinoa mixture, pressing gently to pack it in.

7. Place the stuffed mushrooms on the prepared baking sheet and bake in the preheated oven for 15-20 minutes, or until the mushrooms are tender and the filling is heated through.

8. Once cooked, remove the stuffed mushrooms from the oven and let them cool slightly before serving.

9. Serve the quinoa stuffed mushrooms hot, garnished with additional chopped parsley and lemon wedges if desired.

Enjoy these Quinoa Stuffed Mushrooms as a delicious and nutritious appetizer or side dish that's perfect for supporting overall health during menopause. They're packed with protein, fiber, vitamins, and minerals from the quinoa and vegetables, making them an excellent choice for women following the Galveston Diet.

64. Turkey and vegetable stir-fry with ginger sauce

Ingredients:

For the Stir-Fry:

- 1 pound turkey breast, thinly sliced
- 2 tablespoons olive oil or sesame oil
- 2 cups mixed vegetables

(such as bell peppers, broccoli, snap peas, carrots, mushrooms)

- 2 cloves garlic, minced
- 1 tablespoon grated ginger
- Salt and pepper to taste
- Cooked quinoa or brown rice, for serving

For the Ginger Sauce:

- 1/4 cup low-sodium soy sauce or tamari
- 2 tablespoons rice vinegar
- 1 tablespoon honey or maple syrup
- 1 tablespoon sesame oil
- 1 tablespoon grated ginger
- 1 teaspoon cornstarch (optional, for thickening)

Instructions:

1. In a small bowl, whisk together all the ingredients for the ginger sauce: soy sauce or tamari, rice vinegar, honey or maple syrup, sesame oil, and grated ginger. If you prefer a thicker sauce, whisk in cornstarch until dissolved. Set aside.

2. Heat 1 tablespoon of olive oil or sesame oil in a large skillet or wok over medium-high heat. Add the thinly sliced turkey breast and stir-fry until cooked through, about 5-7 minutes. Remove the turkey from the skillet and set aside.

3. In the same skillet or wok, heat the remaining tablespoon of oil over medium-high heat. Add the mixed vegetables and stir-fry for 5-7 minutes, or until they are crisp-tender.

4. Add the minced garlic and grated ginger to the skillet with the vegetables and stir-fry for another 1-2 minutes until fragrant.

5. Return the cooked turkey to the skillet with the vegetables.

6. Pour the ginger sauce over the turkey and vegetables in the skillet. Stir well to coat everything evenly in the sauce.

7. Cook for an additional 2-3 minutes, or until the sauce has thickened slightly and everything is heated through.

8. Season with salt and pepper to taste. Serve the turkey and vegetable stir-fry hot over cooked quinoa or brown rice.

Enjoy this delicious and nutritious Turkey and Vegetable Stir-Fry with Ginger Sauce as a satisfying meal that's perfect for supporting overall health during menopause.

This recipe provides lean protein, fiber, vitamins, minerals, and anti-inflammatory properties from the turkey, vegetables, and ginger, making it an excellent choice for women following the Galveston Diet. Enjoy!

65. Greek yogurt with cucumber and dill

Ingredients:
- 1 cup Greek yogurt (low-fat or full-fat, according to preference)
- 1/2 cucumber, grated and squeezed to remove excess moisture
- 1 tablespoon chopped fresh dill
- 1 clove garlic, minced (optional)
- 1 tablespoon lemon juice
- Salt and pepper to taste

Instructions:

1. In a mixing bowl, combine the Greek yogurt, grated cucumber, chopped fresh dill, minced garlic (if using), lemon juice, salt, and pepper. Mix well until all ingredients are evenly incorporated.

2. Taste and adjust seasoning with more salt, pepper, or lemon juice if needed.

3. Transfer the Greek yogurt mixture to a serving bowl. Garnish with a sprig of fresh dill or a slice of cucumber, if desired.

4. Serve the Greek yogurt with cucumber and dill immediately as a refreshing dip or spread.

Enjoy this delicious and nutritious Greek Yogurt with Cucumber and Dill as a satisfying snack or appetizer that's perfect for supporting overall health during menopause.

This recipe provides protein, probiotics, vitamins, minerals, and anti-inflammatory properties from the Greek yogurt, cucumber, and dill, making it an excellent choice for women following the Galveston Diet.

66. Eggplant lasagna with ricotta and spinach

Ingredients:
- 2 medium eggplants, thinly sliced lengthwise
- Olive oil, for brushing
- Salt and pepper to taste

For the Ricotta and Spinach Filling:
- 1/2 cup grated Parmesan cheese
- 1 large egg
- 2 cloves garlic, minced
- 1 teaspoon dried oregano
- 1 teaspoon dried basil
- Salt and pepper to taste
- 1 cup chopped spinach, fresh or frozen (thawed and drained)
- 2 cups ricotta cheese (low-fat or full-fat, according to preference)

For the Tomato Sauce:
- 2 cups marinara sauce (store-bought or homemade)
- 2 cloves garlic, minced
- 1 teaspoon dried oregano
- 1 teaspoon dried basil
- Salt and pepper to taste

For Assembly:
- 1 cup shredded mozzarella cheese
- Fresh basil leaves, chopped, for garnish (optional)

Instructions:

1. Preheat your oven to 375°F (190°C). Line two baking sheets with parchment paper.

2. Place the thinly sliced eggplant on the prepared baking sheets in a single layer. Brush both sides of the eggplant slices with olive oil and season with salt and pepper.

3. Roast the eggplant slices in the preheated oven for 15-20 minutes, or until they are tender and slightly golden. Remove from the oven and set aside.

4. While the eggplant is roasting, prepare the ricotta and spinach filling. In a mixing bowl, combine the ricotta cheese, chopped spinach, grated Parmesan cheese, egg, minced garlic, dried oregano, dried basil, salt, and pepper. Mix until well combined. Set aside.

5. In a separate saucepan, heat the marinara sauce over medium heat. Add the minced garlic, dried oregano, dried basil, salt, and pepper. Simmer for 5-10 minutes to allow the flavors to meld. Remove from heat and set aside.

6. To assemble the lasagna, spread a thin layer of tomato sauce on the bottom of a baking dish.

7. Arrange a layer of roasted eggplant slices on top of the tomato sauce. Spread half of the ricotta and spinach filling over the eggplant slices.

8. Repeat the layers: tomato sauce, eggplant slices, remaining ricotta and spinach filling.

9. Top the lasagna with a final layer of roasted eggplant slices. Spread the remaining tomato sauce over the top. Sprinkle shredded mozzarella cheese evenly over the top of the lasagna.

10. Cover the baking dish with aluminum foil and bake in the preheated oven for 25-30 minutes.

11. Remove the foil and continue baking for an additional 10-15 minutes, or until the cheese is melted and bubbly.

12. Once cooked, remove the lasagna from the oven and let it rest for a few minutes before slicing. Garnish with chopped fresh basil leaves, if desired, before serving.

Enjoy this delicious and nutritious Eggplant Lasagna with Ricotta and Spinach as a satisfying meal that's perfect for supporting overall health during menopause.

This recipe provides fiber, protein, vitamins, minerals, and anti-inflammatory properties from the eggplant, spinach, ricotta cheese, and herbs, making it an excellent choice for women following the Galveston Diet.

67. Lentil and sweet potato curry

Ingredients:

- 1 cup dry lentils (brown or green), rinsed and drained
- 2 medium sweet potatoes, peeled and diced
- 1 tablespoon olive oil or coconut oil
- 1 onion, diced
- 3 cloves garlic, minced
- 1 tablespoon grated ginger
- 1 tablespoon curry powder
- 1 teaspoon ground cumin
- 1 teaspoon ground coriander
- 1/4 teaspoon cayenne pepper (optional, for heat)
- 1 (14 oz) can coconut milk
- 1/2 teaspoon turmeric powder
- 1 (14 oz) can diced tomatoes
- 2 cups vegetable broth
- Salt and pepper to taste
- Fresh cilantro leaves, chopped, for garnish (optional)
- Cooked brown rice or quinoa, for serving

Instructions:

1. In a large pot or Dutch oven, heat the olive oil over medium heat. Add the diced onion and cook until softened, about 5 minutes.

2. Add the minced garlic and grated ginger to the pot and cook for another 1-2 minutes until fragrant.

3. Stir in the curry powder, ground cumin, ground coriander, turmeric powder, and cayenne pepper (if using). Cook for another minute until the spices are aromatic.

4. Add the rinsed lentils, diced sweet potatoes, coconut milk, diced tomatoes (with their juices), and vegetable broth to the pot. Stir well to combine.

5. Bring the mixture to a boil, then reduce the heat to low. Cover and simmer for 25-30 minutes, or until the lentils and sweet potatoes are tender and the curry has thickened.

6. Season with salt and pepper to taste. If the curry is too thick, you can add more vegetable broth or water to reach your desired consistency.

7. Once cooked, remove the pot from the heat and let the curry rest for a few minutes before serving.

8. Serve the lentil and sweet potato curry hot over cooked brown rice or quinoa. Garnish with chopped fresh cilantro leaves, if desired.

Enjoy this delicious and nutritious Lentil and Sweet Potato Curry as a satisfying meal that's perfect for supporting overall health during menopause.

This recipe provides fiber, plant-based protein, vitamins, minerals, and anti-inflammatory properties from the lentils, sweet potatoes, and aromatic spices, making it an excellent choice for women following the Galveston Diet. Enjoy!

68. Grilled chicken Caesar salad with homemade dressing

Ingredients:
For the Grilled Chicken:
- 2 boneless, skinless chicken breasts
- 2 tablespoons olive oil
- 2 cloves garlic, minced
- 1 teaspoon dried oregano
- Salt and pepper to taste

For the Salad:
- 1 large head of romaine lettuce, chopped
- 1 cup cherry tomatoes, halved
- 1/4 cup grated Parmesan cheese
- Croutons (optional)

For the Caesar Dressing:
- 1/2 cup Greek yogurt
- 2 tablespoons grated Parmesan cheese
- 2 tablespoons lemon juice
- 1 tablespoon Dijon mustard
- 1 clove garlic, minced
- 1 teaspoon Worcestershire sauce
- 1 teaspoon anchovy paste (optional)
- Salt and pepper to taste

Instructions:

1. Preheat your grill to medium-high heat.

2. In a small bowl, whisk together the olive oil, minced garlic, dried oregano, salt, and pepper. Brush the mixture over the chicken breasts, coating them evenly.

3. Grill the chicken breasts for 6-8 minutes per side, or until they are cooked through and no longer pink in the center. Remove from the grill and let them rest for a few minutes before slicing.

4. While the chicken is grilling, prepare the Caesar dressing. In a mixing bowl, combine the Greek yogurt, grated Parmesan cheese, lemon juice, Dijon mustard, minced garlic, Worcestershire sauce, anchovy paste (if using), salt, and pepper. Whisk until smooth and well combined. Adjust seasoning to taste.

5. Once the chicken has rested, slice it into thin strips.

6. In a large salad bowl, combine the chopped romaine lettuce, cherry tomatoes, and grated Parmesan cheese.

7. Add the sliced grilled chicken to the salad bowl. Drizzle the Caesar dressing over the salad and toss until everything is evenly coated.

8. Serve the grilled chicken Caesar salad immediately, garnished with croutons if desired.

Enjoy this delicious and nutritious Grilled Chicken Caesar Salad with Homemade Dressing as a satisfying meal that's perfect for supporting overall health during menopause.

This recipe provides lean protein, fiber, vitamins, minerals, and anti-inflammatory properties from the grilled chicken, romaine lettuce, tomatoes, and Greek yogurt-based dressing, making it an excellent choice for women following the Galveston Diet.

69. Tofu and vegetable stir-fry with cashews

Ingredients:
For the Stir-Fry:
- 14 oz (400g) firm tofu, pressed and cubed
- 2 tablespoons soy sauce or tamari
- 2 tablespoons sesame oil, divided
- 1 tablespoon cornstarch
- 1 tablespoon olive oil or coconut oil
- 2 cloves garlic, minced
- 1 tablespoon grated ginger
- 1 red bell pepper, thinly sliced
- 1 yellow bell pepper, thinly sliced
- 1 cup broccoli florets
- 1 cup snap peas or snow peas
- 1 medium carrot, julienned
- 1/2 cup unsalted cashews
- Cooked brown rice or quinoa, for serving

For the Sauce:
- 1/4 cup low-sodium soy sauce or tamari
- 2 tablespoons rice vinegar
- 1 tablespoon honey or maple syrup
- 1 tablespoon sesame oil
- 1 teaspoon cornstarch
- 1/4 cup water

Instructions:

1. In a bowl, combine the cubed tofu, soy sauce or tamari, and 1 tablespoon of sesame oil. Toss gently to coat the tofu evenly. Allow it to marinate for about 15-20 minutes.

2. In the meantime, prepare the sauce by whisking together all the sauce ingredients in a small bowl until the cornstarch is fully dissolved. Set aside.

3. Heat the remaining tablespoon of sesame oil and olive oil (or coconut oil) in a large skillet or wok over medium-high heat. Add the marinated tofu cubes (reserving any excess marinade) and cook until golden brown on all sides, about 5-7 minutes. Remove the tofu from the skillet and set it aside.

4. In the same skillet, add the minced garlic and grated ginger. Sauté for about 1 minute until fragrant.

5. Add the sliced bell peppers, broccoli florets, snap peas (or snow peas), and julienned carrots to the skillet. Cook, stirring frequently, for about 5-7 minutes, or until the vegetables are tender-crisp.

6. Return the cooked tofu to the skillet. Add the unsalted cashews and the reserved marinade. Stir well to combine.

7. Give the sauce a quick stir to recombine, then pour it over the tofu and vegetables in the skillet.

8. Continue to cook for another 2-3 minutes, or until the sauce has thickened and everything is heated through. Taste and adjust seasoning if necessary.

9. Serve the tofu and vegetable stir-fry hot over cooked brown rice or quinoa.

70. Quinoa salad with roasted butternut squash and cranberries

Ingredients:
For the Salad:
- 1 cup quinoa, rinsed
- 2 cups water or vegetable broth
- 1 small butternut squash, peeled, seeded, and diced into small cubes
- 2 tablespoons olive oil
- 1 teaspoon ground cinnamon
- Salt and pepper to taste

- 1/2 cup dried cranberries
- 1/4 cup chopped fresh parsley or cilantro
- 1/4 cup chopped walnuts or pecans (optional)

For the Dressing:
- 3 tablespoons extra virgin olive oil
- 2 tablespoons apple cider vinegar or balsamic vinegar
- 1 tablespoon maple syrup or honey
- 1 teaspoon Dijon mustard
- Salt and pepper to taste

Instructions:

1. Preheat your oven to 400°F (200°C).

2. In a medium saucepan, combine the quinoa and water or vegetable broth. Bring to a boil, then reduce the heat to low, cover, and simmer for 15-20 minutes, or until the quinoa is cooked and the liquid is absorbed. Remove from heat and let it cool.

3. While the quinoa is cooking, spread the diced butternut squash in a single layer on a baking sheet. Drizzle with olive oil and sprinkle with ground cinnamon, salt, and pepper. Toss to coat evenly.

4. Roast the butternut squash in the preheated oven for 20-25 minutes, or until tender and lightly caramelized. Remove from the oven and let it cool slightly.

5. In a small bowl, whisk together the ingredients for the dressing: extra virgin olive oil, apple cider vinegar or balsamic vinegar, maple syrup or honey, Dijon mustard, salt, and pepper. Set aside.

6. In a large mixing bowl, combine the cooked quinoa, roasted butternut squash, dried cranberries, chopped parsley or cilantro, and chopped walnuts or pecans (if using).

7. Pour the dressing over the quinoa salad and toss gently to coat everything evenly. Taste and adjust seasoning with more salt and pepper if needed.

8. Serve the quinoa salad with roasted butternut squash and cranberries at room temperature or chilled.

Enjoy this delicious and nutritious Quinoa Salad with Roasted Butternut Squash and Cranberries as a satisfying meal that's perfect for supporting overall health during menopause

71. Turkey and black bean chili

Ingredients:
- 1 tablespoon olive oil
- 1 pound ground turkey
- 1 onion, chopped
- 3 cloves garlic, minced
- 1 red bell pepper, chopped
- 1 green bell pepper, chopped
- 1 jalapeño pepper, seeded and finely chopped (optional, for heat)
- 1 tablespoon chili powder
- 1 teaspoon ground cumin
- 1 teaspoon dried oregano
- 1/2 teaspoon smoked paprika
- 1/4 teaspoon cayenne pepper (optional, for extra heat)
- Salt and pepper to taste
- 2 (15 oz) cans black beans, rinsed and drained
- 1 (14.5 oz) can diced tomatoes
- 1 cup low-sodium chicken broth or vegetable broth
- 1/4 cup chopped fresh cilantro, for garnish (optional)
- Greek yogurt or sour cream, for serving (optional)
- Sliced green onions, for garnish (optional)
- Lime wedges, for serving (optional)

Instructions:

1. Heat the olive oil in a large pot or Dutch oven over medium heat. Add the ground turkey and cook, breaking it up with a spoon, until browned and cooked through.

2. Add the chopped onion, minced garlic, chopped red bell pepper, chopped green bell pepper, and chopped jalapeño pepper (if using) to the pot. Cook, stirring occasionally, until the vegetables are softened, about 5-7 minutes.

3. Stir in the chili powder, ground cumin, dried oregano, smoked paprika, cayenne pepper (if using), salt, and pepper. Cook for another minute until the spices are fragrant.

4. Add the rinsed and drained black beans, diced tomatoes (with their juices), and chicken broth to the pot. Stir well to combine.

5. Bring the chili to a simmer, then reduce the heat to low. Cover and let it simmer for 20-30 minutes, stirring occasionally, to allow the flavors to meld and the chili to thicken.

6. Taste and adjust seasoning with more salt and pepper if needed.

7. Serve the turkey and black bean chili hot, garnished with chopped fresh cilantro, Greek yogurt or sour cream, sliced green onions, and lime wedges if desired.

Enjoy this delicious and nutritious Turkey and Black Bean Chili as a comforting meal that's perfect for supporting overall health during menopause.

This recipe provides lean protein, fiber, vitamins, minerals, and anti-inflammatory properties from the turkey, black beans, and a variety of vegetables and spices, making it an excellent choice for women following the Galveston Diet. Enjoy!

72. Greek yogurt with mango and coconut flakes

Ingredients:
- 1 cup Greek yogurt (low-fat or full-fat, according to preference)
- 1 ripe mango, peeled, pitted, and diced
- 2 tablespoons unsweetened coconut flakes

Instructions:

1. In a serving bowl or glass, add the Greek yogurt.

2. Top the Greek yogurt with the diced mango.

3. Sprinkle the unsweetened coconut flakes over the mango and yogurt.

4. Serve immediately and enjoy!

This Greek Yogurt with Mango and Coconut Flakes is not only delicious but also provides a balance of protein, healthy fats, and natural sweetness from the mango. It's a satisfying and nutritious snack or dessert option that's perfect for supporting overall health during menopause

Thank you